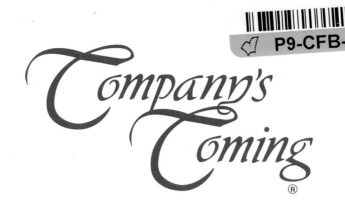

Company's Coming®

30-Minute Diabetic Cooking

Jean Paré

www.companyscoming.com
visit our website

Front Cover

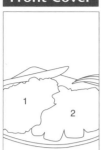

1. Feta Ruby Chard, page 138
2. Raspberry Steak, page 68

Props courtesy of: Casa Bugatti

Back Cover

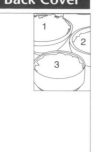

1. Mango Chutney Steak Salad, page 30
2. Orange Quinoa Salad, page 34
3. Tropical Shrimp Fruit Salad, page 37

Props courtesy of: Cherison Enterprises Inc.

We gratefully acknowledge the following suppliers for their generous support of our Test and Photography Kitchens:

Broil King Barbecues   *Hamilton Beach® Canada*   *Proctor Silex® Canada*
Corelle®   *Lagostina®*   *Tupperware®*

30-Minute Diabetic Cooking

First Printing October 2008

Library and Archives Canada Cataloguing in Publication
Paré, Jean, date
30-minute diabetic cooking / Jean Paré.
(Original series)
Includes index.
At head of title: Company's coming.
ISBN 978-1-897069-79-0
1. Diabetes—Diet therapy—Recipes. 2. Quick and easy cookery. I. Title.
II. Title: Thirty-minute diabetic cooking. III. Series: Paré, Jean, date.
Original series.
RC662.P38 2008   641.5'6314   C2008-901561-4

Published by
Company's Coming Publishing Limited
2311 – 96 Street
Edmonton, Alberta, Canada T6N 1G3
Tel: 780-450-6223   Fax: 780-450-1857
www.companyscoming.com

Company's Coming is a registered trademark owned by
Company's Coming Publishing Limited

We acknowledge the financial support of the Government of Canada through the Book Publishing Industry Development Program (BPIDP) for our publishing activities.

Printed in China

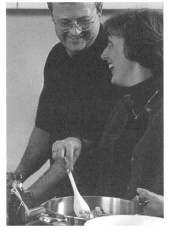

Company's Coming Cookbooks

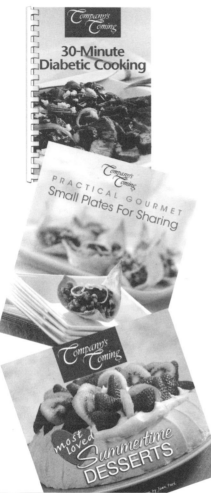

Original Series

- Softcover, 160 pages
- 6" x 9" (15 cm x 23 cm) format
- Lay-flat plastic comb binding
- Full-colour photos
- Nutrition information

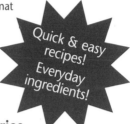

Quick & easy recipes! Everyday ingredients!

Practical Gourmet Series

- Hardcover, 224 pages
- 8" x 10" (21 cm x 26 cm) format
- Full-colour throughout
- Nutrition information

Most Loved Recipe Collection

- Hardcover, 128 pages
- 8 3/4" x 8 3/4" (22 cm x 22 cm) format
- Durable sewn binding
- Full-colour throughout
- Nutrition information

Special Occasion Series

- Softcover, 176 pages
- 8 1/2" x 11" (22 cm x 28 cm) format
- Full-colour throughout
- Nutrition information

See page 157 for more cookbooks.
For a complete listing, visit
www.companyscoming.com

Table of Contents

Breakfast,
Brunch & Lunch

Soups & Salads

Snacks &
Smoothies

Beef & Pork

Chicken &
Turkey

Fish & Seafood

Meatless

Sides

Desserts

The Company's Coming Story

Jean Paré (pronounced "jeen PAIR-ee") grew up understanding that the combination of family, friends and home cooking is the best recipe for a good life. From her mother, she learned to appreciate good cooking, while her father praised even her earliest attempts in the kitchen. When Jean left home, she took with her a love of cooking, many family recipes and an intriguing desire to read cookbooks as if they were novels!

"Never share a recipe you wouldn't use yourself."

When her four children had all reached school age, Jean volunteered to cater the 50th anniversary celebration of the Vermilion School of Agriculture, now Lakeland College, in Alberta, Canada. Working out of her home, Jean prepared a dinner for more than 1,000 people, launching a flourishing catering operation that continued for over 18 years. During that time, she had countless opportunities to test new ideas with immediate feedback— resulting in empty plates and contented customers! Whether preparing cocktail sandwiches for a house party or serving a hot meal for 1,500 people, Jean Paré earned a reputation for great food, courteous service and reasonable prices.

As requests for her recipes increased, Jean was often asked the question, "Why don't you write a cookbook?" Jean responded by teaming up with her son, Grant Lovig, in the fall of 1980 to form Company's Coming Publishing Limited. The publication of *150 Delicious Squares* on April 14, 1981 marked the debut of what would soon become one of the world's most popular cookbook series.

The company has grown since those early days when Jean worked from a spare bedroom in her home. Today, she continues to write recipes while working closely with the staff of the Recipe Factory, as the Company's Coming test kitchen is affectionately known.

There she fills the role of mentor, assisting with the development of recipes people most want to use for everyday cooking and easy entertaining. Every Company's Coming recipe is kitchen-tested before it is approved for publication.

Jean's daughter, Gail Lovig, is responsible for marketing and distribution, leading a team that includes sales personnel located in major cities across Canada. Company's Coming cookbooks are distributed in Canada, the United States, Australia and other world markets. Bestsellers many times over in English, Company's Coming cookbooks have also been published in French and Spanish.

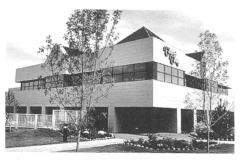

Familiar and trusted in home kitchens around the world, Company's Coming cookbooks are offered in a variety of formats. Highly regarded as kitchen workbooks, the softcover Original Series, with its lay-flat plastic comb binding, is still a favourite among readers.

Jean Paré's approach to cooking has always called for quick and easy recipes using everyday ingredients. That view has served her well. The recipient of many awards, including the Queen Elizabeth Golden Jubilee Medal, Jean was appointed Member of the Order of Canada, her country's highest lifetime achievement honour.

Jean continues to gain new supporters by adhering to what she calls The Golden Rule of Cooking: *Never share a recipe you wouldn't use yourself.* It's an approach that has worked—millions of times over!

Foreword

It's a fact—diet is a key factor in managing diabetes. But these days, healthy eating is something that everyone should be concerned with. Properly portioning meals and monitoring intake of fat, salt and sugar are part of how many people live. Diabetic cooking isn't just for those with diabetes or their families; it's a healthy, balanced way to eat that all people can benefit from.

Before we started developing *30-Minute Diabetic Cooking*, we met with a focus group to find out what would be most helpful in a diabetic cookbook. The group talked about ingredients to avoid, the kinds of recipes that best suit their requirements and the need for adequate information to help them in portioning meals. But what was the most universally agreed upon request? Recipes that can be prepared quickly!

What we have created is a cookbook suitable for those with diabetes and their families. We've given you great-tasting recipes for breakfasts, lunches, dinners, desserts and snacks. The recipes were written for a busy lifestyle, so they're practical and quick to put together—ready in 30 minutes or less! We've also given you tips for diabetic eating and hints for quick and easy cooking.

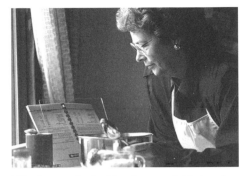

Whether you're looking for a portable lunch like Toasted Chicken Caesar Sandwiches, a satisfying snack like the Tropical Tango Tofu Smoothie or a hearty serving of the Pork Apple Skillet as a main course, you're sure to find plenty of nutritious options. And because everyone needs to have at least a little chocolate to keep things fun, be sure to try the Triple-Chocolate Shortcakes in our Desserts section.

So if you're cooking for yourself or a family member with diabetes, or just wanting to eat healthier, you'll be sure to find great-tasting, nutritious meal options that are super-speedy to prepare in *30-Minute Diabetic Cooking!*

Jean Paré

Nutrition Information Guidelines

Each recipe is analyzed using the most current version of the Canadian Nutrient File from Health Canada, which is based on the United States Department of Agriculture (USDA) Nutrient Database.

- If more than one ingredient is listed (such as "butter or hard margarine"), or if a range is given (1 – 2 tsp., 5 – 10 mL), only the first ingredient or first amount is analyzed.

- For meat, poultry and fish, the serving size per person is based on the recommended 4 oz. (113 g) uncooked weight (without bone), which is 2 – 3 oz. (57 – 85 g) cooked weight (without bone)—approximately the size of a deck of playing cards.

- Milk used is 1% M.F. (milk fat), unless otherwise stated.

- Cooking oil used is canola oil, unless otherwise stated.

- Ingredients indicating "sprinkle," "optional," or "for garnish" are not included in the nutrition information.

- The fat in recipes and combination foods can vary greatly depending on the sources and types of fats used in each specific ingredient. For these reasons, the amount of saturated, monounsaturated and polyunsaturated fats may not add up to the total fat content.

Vera C. Mazurak, Ph.D.
Nutritionist

About Diabetes

Diabetes, in the most general terms, is caused when someone has too much glucose in their blood because the body isn't processing it properly. This glucose comes from the food we consume, specifically from the digestion of carbohydrates like grains, fruits and vegetables. For most people, the pancreas produces enough insulin to break down glucose, which enables the body to use it as energy.

For individuals with Type 1 diabetes, insulin injections are required to break down glucose. This is because their bodies are producing very little insulin, or perhaps none at all. For those with Type 2 diabetes, insulin injections are generally not required as these people's bodies are able to produce some insulin. These individuals may be able to mange their diabetes with diet alone, or by using a combination of diet and medication.

Diabetic eating

Managing diabetes with a proper diet is imperative. Every person with diabetes needs to consult with a doctor or dietitian to determine an appropriate eating plan, but here are a few tips to consider:

Choosing ingredients wisely

The world is a changing place. People are becoming more and more aware of health issues and are making smarter choices about what they eat. Using ingredients with lower levels of fat, sugar and salt will help you to achieve your dietary goals.

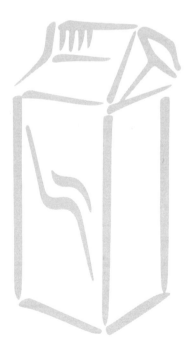

Choosing leaner cuts of meat and lower-fat dairy products are just a few examples of ways you can make your cooking more nutritious. Also, it can be helpful to choose fats that have some nutritional benefit. Try using tub margarines that contain no trans-fats, or choose canola oil or cooking spray for frying.

Of course, how you cook your meals also makes a difference. Trim fat from your meat before cooking and use cooking methods such as grilling, poaching, baking and stir-frying to limit the amount of unwanted fat you are adding to your food.

Making smarter choices

Although ingredients like salt, fat, alcohol and sugar can make food taste better, the benefit doesn't necessarily justify the effects on your health. The same can be said about convenience foods. Although convenience foods often save on time, they are often so high in fat, salt and sugar that they just aren't worth it. Of course, this doesn't mean that you'll have to suffer through a boring diet of flavourless food or meals that take forever to prepare. It just means making smarter choices about what you are going to eat.

Choose fresh fruits and vegetables that are in season to help limit the expense. Using recipes that are quick and easy helps to reduce the amount of time you'll spend in the kitchen. Try making larger batches of foods that can be portioned and reheated later so you don't have to turn to unhealthy convenience foods when you're in a rush.

Stock up on snacks

Eating smaller quantities of food more often helps to prevent blood sugar spikes. Having lots of convenient little snacks on hand will help to fill the gaps between meals. Ensure these snacks are nutritious and low in fat. Be sure to keep some portable snacks on hand, too—this way you will always have something you can grab on your way out the door or pack in your lunch.

Everything in moderation

The best carbohydrates are the complex carbs found in unprocessed foods, like vegetables or whole grains. They're a great source of energy and they contain lots of fibre and nutrients, too. However, there are no forbidden foods in a diabetic diet. Everyone needs a special treat once in awhile, so allowing yourself a small piece of chocolate or candy will keep you from feeling like you're giving up the foods you enjoy most. Moderating your intake of sweets and starchy carbohydrates will help you to keep your blood sugar manageable.

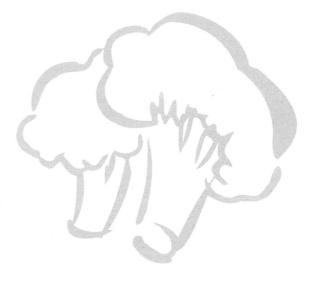

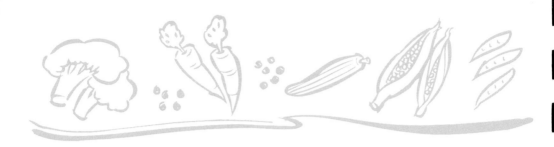

Diabetic Choices (Beyond the Basics)

Tracking what you're eating is imperative for a diabetic diet. Each recipe in *30-Minute Diabetic Cooking* includes a basic breakdown of nutritional information, as well as diabetic choice values for the Beyond the Basics meal-planning guide. Beyond the Basics groups together foods that are similar in carbohydrate content. The names of the categories have been changed to better reflect the foods in the group. For example, Starches has become Grains and Starches, whereas Sugars has become Other Choices to better reflect the sweets and snack foods within this group. Although the serving size of each food within a particular group may vary, one serving of each food in that group will have the same approximate composition of carbohydrates, protein, fat and calories. If no choices are listed, it means that the serving size suggested for that recipe does not contain enough carbohydrates to constitute a choice in any category.

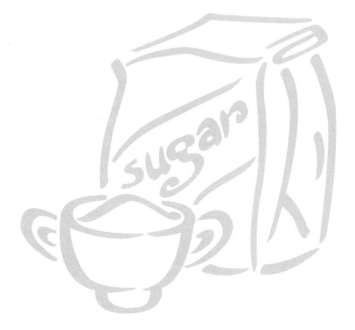

For people on insulin who require precise carbohydrate counting, the nutritional information provides a useful guideline for total grams of carbohydrate and

Tips for Timely Cooking

Sure, everyone wants to eat better, but who has the time to do all that cooking? Here are a few tips that will help you to make the most of your time in the kitchen:

Planning ahead

It's a lot easier to attain a goal if you plan for it. This is also true of managing your eating. Making a weekly meal plan helps you save time in so many ways. You will have an easier time with grocery shopping if you know ahead of time what you're going to need and make a list. And you'll come home from work every evening knowing what's on the menu, so you won't have to waste time looking around your kitchen for inspiration.

Keeping high-demand items in stock

Keeping the essentials on hand is always helpful. Keep a ready supply of ingredients you use often. This can include pantry items like flour, tomato sauce or dried lentils and freezer items like frozen veggies or lean meat. When your stock starts to dwindle, just add the item to your grocery list and replenish the supply on your next shopping trip. Keeping your kitchen well-stocked is a great time saver and helps to eliminate emergency trips to the grocery store.

Doubling up

Make your freezer your best friend. You can cook larger amounts of grains in advance and freeze them in smaller portions for recipes that use them. This is especially handy for those grains that take a long time to cook, such as wild rice. You can also pre-cook and freeze chicken, ground beef or beans to cut the cooking time later. Making big batches of recipes that freeze well, then portioning and storing them for busier days, is also a great way to make sure a nutritious meal is never out of reach, even when time is a precious commodity.

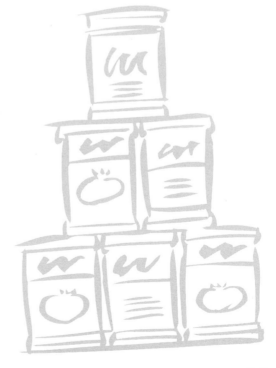

11

Oven Pancake

Make one big pancake in the oven as a convenient alternative to frying several smaller ones. Sandwich wedges of this dense cake with yogurt, cheese or peanut butter.

Canola oil	1/2 tsp.	2 mL
All-purpose flour	1/2 cup	125 mL
Quick-cooking rolled oats	3 tbsp.	50 mL
Brown sugar, packed	2 tbsp.	30 mL
Baking powder	1 tsp.	5 mL
Ground cinnamon	1/2 tsp.	2 mL
Salt, just a pinch		
Large egg	1	1
Milk	3/4 cup	175 mL
Canola oil	1 tsp.	5 mL
Vanilla extract	1/2 tsp.	2 mL
Dried cranberries	1/4 cup	60 mL

Preheat oven to 450°F (230°C). Heat first amount of canola oil in large frying pan on medium.

Combine next 6 ingredients in medium bowl. Make a well in centre.

Whisk next 4 ingredients in small bowl. Add to well. Stir until just combined.

Scatter cranberries on bottom of frying pan. Pour batter over top. Immediately swirl batter to coat bottom, lifting and tilting pan to ensure entire bottom is covered. Bake on bottom rack in oven (see Tip, page 26) for 15 to 20 minutes until golden and centre springs back when pressed. Gently loosen sides and bottom of pancake with spatula. Carefully transfer to cutting board or plate. Cuts into 4 wedges. Serves 2.

1 serving: 343 Calories; 7.4 g Total Fat (3.5 g Mono, 1.4 g Poly, 1.6 g Sat); 99 mg Cholesterol; 60 g Carbohydrate; 2 g Fibre; 11 g Protein; 214 mg Sodium

CHOICES: 2 Grains & Starches; 1 Other Choices; 1/2 Meat & Alternatives; 1/2 Fats

Apple Barley Porridge

When it comes to nutritious breakfasts, oatmeal's always been the top choice—until now! This hearty porridge includes the goodness of flaxseed and barley with the classic, comforting flavours of apple and cinnamon.

Water	2 1/2 cups	625 mL
Large flake rolled oats	1 1/2 cups	375 mL
Cooked pot barley (about 1 cup, 250 mL, uncooked)	2 cups	500 mL
Flaxseed	1 tbsp.	15 mL
Ground cinnamon	1/2 tsp.	2 mL
Salt	1/4 tsp.	1 mL
Unsweetened applesauce	1 cup	250 mL
Brown sugar, packed	1 tbsp.	15 mL

Bring water to a boil in medium saucepan. Reduce heat to medium-low. Add oats. Stir.

Add next 4 ingredients. Stir. Simmer, covered, for about 10 minutes, stirring occasionally, until oats are tender.

Add applesauce and brown sugar. Cook and stir for about 1 minute until heated through. Makes about 6 cups (1.5 L). Serves 6.

1 serving: 182 Calories; 2.5 g Total Fat (trace Mono, 0.1 g Poly, 0.1 g Sat); 0 mg Cholesterol; 35 g Carbohydrate; 5 g Fibre; 5 g Protein; 101 mg Sodium

CHOICES: 1 1/2 Grains & Starches

Paré Pointer

After tasting his cough medicine, he said he would rather have the cough.

Orzo Sausage Bake

For cold-weather comfort food, look no further! This spicy, hearty casserole is perfect for lunch or brunch and has a texture that's halfway between stuffing and savoury bread pudding.

Water	8 cups	2 L
Salt	1 tsp.	5 mL
Orzo	1 cup	250 mL
Canola oil	1 tsp.	5 mL
Hot Italian sausage, casing removed	3/4 lb.	340 g
Chopped onion	1 cup	250 mL
Grated part-skim mozzarella cheese	1 1/2 cups	375 mL
Light ricotta cheese	1 cup	250 mL
Fine dry bread crumbs	1/2 cup	125 mL
Italian seasoning	1 tsp.	5 mL
Paprika	1/2 tsp.	2 mL

Preheat oven to 425°F (220°C). Combine water and salt in large saucepan. Bring to a boil. Add pasta. Boil, uncovered, for 8 to 10 minutes, stirring occasionally, until tender but firm. Drain. Return to same pot. Cover to keep warm.

Meanwhile, heat canola oil in large frying pan on medium-high. Add sausage and onion. Scramble-fry for about 5 minutes until sausage is browned. Drain. Add to pasta. Stir.

Add next 4 ingredients. Stir. Transfer to greased 2 quart (2 L) baking dish.

Sprinkle with paprika. Bake, uncovered, for about 15 minutes until browned and heated through. Makes about 6 cups (1.5 L). Serves 6.

1 serving: 383 Calories; 16.7 g Total Fat (5.7 g Mono, 1.5 g Poly, 7.5 g Sat); 46 mg Cholesterol; 35 g Carbohydrate; 2 g Fibre; 22 g Protein; 625 mg Sodium

CHOICES: 1 1/2 Grains & Starches; 2 Meat & Alternatives

Bacon Bean Bowl

Eating healthy doesn't have to be unpleasant—sometimes it's okay to compromise. This hearty stew includes a little bacon for flavour and a lot of spinach and beans for added fibre and protein.

Bacon slices, chopped	4	4
Chopped onion	1 cup	250 mL
Garlic cloves, minced	2	2
(or 1/2 tsp., 2 mL, powder)		
Sliced fresh white mushrooms	1 cup	250 mL
Can of white kidney beans, rinsed and drained	14 oz.	398 mL
Tiny bow pasta	1 cup	250 mL
Prepared vegetable broth	2 1/2 cups	625 mL
Fresh spinach leaves, lightly packed	6 cups	1.5 L
Grated lemon zest	1 tbsp.	15 mL
Pepper	1/4 tsp.	1 mL

Combine first 4 ingredients in large frying pan on medium-high. Cook for about 5 minutes, stirring often, until onion is softened and starting to brown.

Add next 3 ingredients. Stir. Bring to a boil. Reduce heat to medium-low. Simmer, covered, for about 10 minutes, stirring often, until pasta is tender but firm.

Add remaining 3 ingredients. Heat and stir for about 2 minutes until spinach is wilted. Makes about 5 cups (1.25 L). Serves 4.

1 serving: 440 Calories; 12.3 g Total Fat (4.6 g Mono, 1.2 g Poly, 3.7 g Sat); 15 mg Cholesterol; 66 g Carbohydrate; 8 g Fibre; 18 g Protein; 548 mg Sodium

CHOICES: 3 Grains & Starches; 1 Vegetables; 1 Meat & Alternatives

Pictured on page 18.

Mexican Egg Wraps

Taste buds still asleep? Wake them up with this combination of spicy salsa, Cheddar cheese and eggs nestled in a soft flour tortilla. This is just about the easiest and most delicious breakfast you could make.

Tub margarine	2 tsp.	10 mL
Large eggs	4	4
Salt, sprinkle		
Pepper, sprinkle		
Salsa	1/2 cup	125 mL
Whole-wheat flour tortillas	4	4
(6 inch, 15 cm, diameter)		
Grated light sharp Cheddar cheese	1/4 cup	60 mL
Finely chopped fresh cilantro	1 tsp.	5 mL

Melt margarine in large frying pan on medium. Break eggs, one at a time, into pan. Pierce yolks with fork. Sprinkle with salt and pepper. Cook, covered, for about 3 minutes until set.

Spread 2 tbsp. (30 mL) salsa on each tortilla, leaving 1 inch (2.5 cm) border. Place 1 egg over salsa on each tortilla. Sprinkle with cheese and cilantro. Fold sides over filling. Roll up from bottom to enclose filling. Makes 4 wraps.

1 wrap: 212 Calories; 9.1 g Total Fat (2.9 g Mono, 2.6 g Poly, 2.6 g Sat); 190 mg Cholesterol; 22 g Carbohydrate; 2 g Fibre; 11 g Protein; 486 mg Sodium

CHOICES: 1 Grains & Starches; 1 Meat & Alternatives

Pictured on page 17.

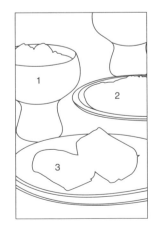

1. Creamy Couscous Parfaits, page 24
2. Waffles With Peanut Butter Spread, page 28
3. Mexican Egg Wraps, above

Props courtesy of: Danesco Inc.

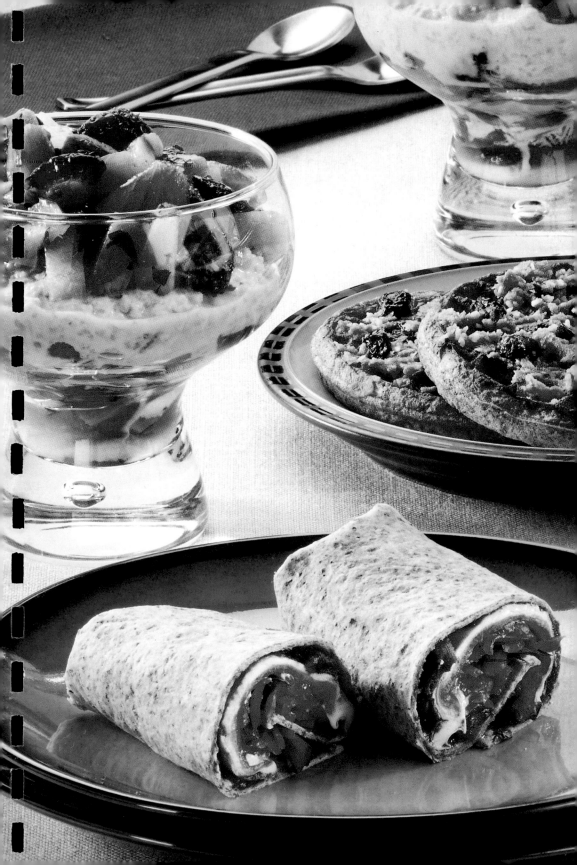

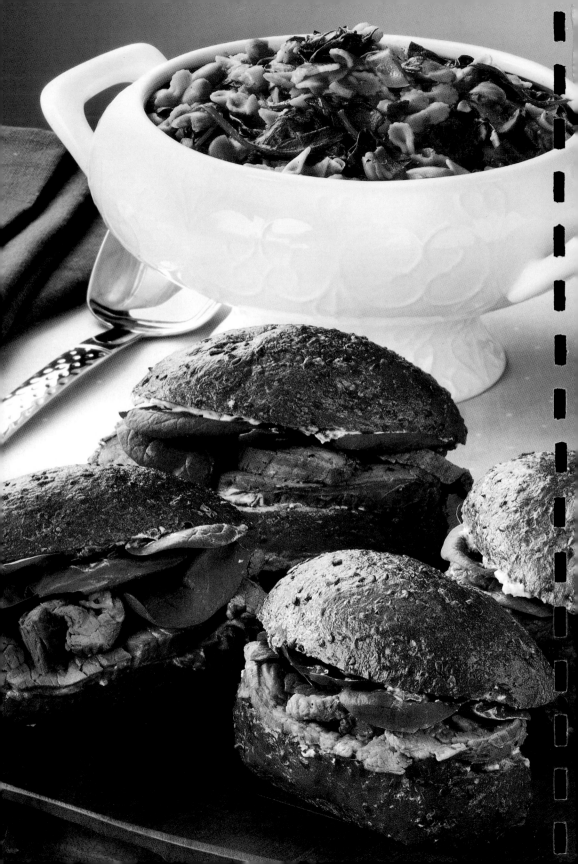

Stylish Steak Sandwiches

A chic twist on a steak and cheese sandwich. Super simple to make at home, but tastes just like it came from a trendy bistro.

Flank steak	3/4 lb.	340 g
Montreal steak spice	1/4 tsp.	1 mL
Chopped roasted red pepper, blotted dry	1/2 cup	125 mL
Light herb and garlic cream cheese	1/3 cup	75 mL
Crusty whole-grain rolls, split	4	4
Montreal steak spice	1/4 tsp.	1 mL
Fresh spinach leaves, lightly packed	2 cups	500 mL

Preheat broiler. Sprinkle both sides of steak with first amount of steak spice. Place on greased baking sheet. Broil on top rack in oven for about 3 minutes per side until desired doneness. Transfer to cutting board. Cover with foil. Let stand for 10 minutes.

Meanwhile, combine red pepper and cream cheese in small bowl. Spread on bun halves.

Thinly slice steak diagonally across the grain. Sprinkle with second amount of steak spice. Arrange beef over cream cheese mixture on each bun. Top with spinach. Set bun tops over spinach. Makes 4 sandwiches.

1 sandwich: 319 Calories; 12.9 g Total Fat (3.6 g Mono, 1.2 g Poly, 5.6 g Sat); 49 mg Cholesterol; 27 g Carbohydrate; 5 g Fibre; 24 g Protein; 557 mg Sodium

CHOICES: 1 Grains & Starches; 2 1/2 Meat & Alternatives

Pictured on page 18.

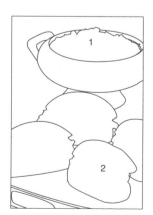

1. Bacon Bean Bowl, page 15
2. Stylish Steak Sandwiches, above

Chipotle Turkey Joes

We're not sure who the famous sloppy joe was named after, but we're sure he'd be proud to have his name attached to this sweet and spicy update to the classic sandwich. Chipotle peppers (pronounced chih-POHT-lay) add some smoky heat.

Canola oil	1 tsp.	5 mL
Ground turkey	3/4 lb.	340 g
Chopped onion	1 cup	250 mL
Chopped roasted red pepper	1/4 cup	60 mL
Garlic cloves, minced	2	2
(or 1/2 tsp., 2 mL, powder)		
Finely chopped chipotle pepper in	1 tsp.	5 mL
adobo sauce (see Tip, page 40)		
Granulated sugar	1 tsp.	5 mL
Ground cumin	1/2 tsp.	2 mL
Ground ginger	1/2 tsp.	2 mL
Salt	1/2 tsp.	2 mL
Pepper	1/4 tsp.	1 mL
All-purpose flour	1 tbsp.	15 mL
Can of diced tomatoes (with juice)	14 oz.	398 mL
Frozen concentrated orange juice	1/4 cup	60 mL
Whole-wheat English muffins, split	4	4

Heat canola oil in large frying pan on medium-high. Add next 10 ingredients. Scramble-fry for about 6 minutes until turkey is no longer pink.

Sprinkle flour over turkey mixture. Heat and stir for 1 minute. Add tomatoes and concentrated orange juice. Stir. Bring to a boil. Reduce heat to medium-low. Simmer, covered, for 5 minutes to blend flavours.

Meanwhile, toast English muffin halves. Place 2 halves on each plate. Spoon turkey mixture over muffin halves. Serves 4.

1 serving: 328 Calories; 3.8 g Total Fat (1.0 g Mono, 0.9 g Poly, 0.3 g Sat); 34 mg Cholesterol; 47 g Carbohydrate; 5 g Fibre; 29 g Protein; 1182 mg Sodium

CHOICES: 1 1/2 Grains & Starches; 1/2 Fruits; 2 Vegetables; 3 Meat & Alternatives

Mandarin Turkey Wraps

Juicy mandarin oranges are truly outstanding in this wholesome wrap of turkey, apple, pecans and cranberries.

Canned mandarin orange segments, drained	1/2 cup	125 mL
Chopped unpeeled tart apple (such as Granny Smith)	1/4 cup	60 mL
Chopped pecans, toasted (see Tip, page 114)	2 tbsp.	30 mL
Dried cranberries	2 tbsp.	30 mL
Non-fat plain yogurt	2 tbsp.	30 mL
Light mayonnaise	1 tbsp.	15 mL
Whole-wheat tortillas (9 inch, 22 cm diameter)	4	4
Lettuce leaves	4	4
Grated part-skim mozzarella cheese	1/2 cup	125 mL
Deli turkey breast slices (about 1/2 lb., 225 g)	8	8

Combine first 6 ingredients in small bowl.

Arrange tortillas on work surface. Layer remaining 3 ingredients, in order given, on each tortilla. Spoon orange mixture along centre of turkey. Fold bottom ends of tortillas over filling. Fold in sides, slightly overlapping, leaving top ends open. Secure with wooden picks. Makes 4 wraps.

1 wrap: 246 Calories; 8.2 g Total Fat (2.9 g Mono, 2.3 g Poly, 2.0 g Sat); 31 mg Cholesterol; 29 g Carbohydrate; 3 g Fibre; 17 g Protein; 819 mg Sodium

CHOICES: 1/2 Grains & Starches; 1/2 Fruits; 2 Meat & Alternatives; 1/2 Fats

Oven Omelette

Can't seem to get the hang of making omelettes in a frying pan?
Try this oven method for quick and tasty results. All of the flavour
with none of the fuss!

Low-cholesterol egg product	1 1/2 cups	375 mL
Finely chopped green onion	2 tbsp.	30 mL
Skim milk	2 tbsp.	30 mL
Salt	1/4 tsp.	1 mL
Pepper	1/8 tsp.	0.5 mL
Cooking spray		
Grated Swiss cheese	1/2 cup	125 mL
Deli turkey breast slices, cut into thin strips	2 oz.	57 g

Preheat oven to 400°F (205°C). Heat 9 x 13 inch (22 x 33 cm) baking dish in oven for 3 minutes. Meanwhile, combine first 5 ingredients in small bowl.

Spray hot baking dish with cooking spray. Pour egg mixture into dish. Bake, uncovered, for about 8 minutes until eggs start to set but are still moist on surface. Cut into 4 pieces.

Sprinkle cheese and turkey onto half of each piece. Bake, uncovered, for about 2 minutes until cheese is melted. Fold omelettes over turkey and cheese. Makes 4 omelettes.

1 omelette: 132 Calories; 5.9 g Total Fat (0 g Mono, 0 g Poly, 2.5 g Sat); 95 mg Cholesterol; 3 g Carbohydrate; trace Fibre; 15 g Protein; 456 mg Sodium

CHOICES: 2 Meat & Alternatives

Paré Pointer

Weather is so colourful—the sun rose and the wind blue.

Thai Beef Lettuce Wraps

Add a taste of Asia to your next lunch. A bold, nutty beef filling is nestled in delicate lettuce leaves for delicious flavour and texture contrasts.

Cooking spray		
Extra-lean ground beef	1 lb.	454 g
Finely grated gingerroot (or 1/4 tsp., 1 mL, ground ginger)	1 tsp.	5 mL
Garlic clove, minced (or 1/4 tsp., 1 mL, powder)	1	1
Diced English cucumber (with peel)	1 1/2 cups	375 mL
Grated carrot	1/2 cup	125 mL
Coarsely chopped fresh basil (or mint), lightly packed	1/4 cup	60 mL
Sweet chili sauce	2 tbsp.	30 mL
Peanut sauce	1/3 cup	75 mL
Hoisin sauce	1 tbsp.	15 mL
Butter lettuce leaves	24	24

Heat large frying pan on medium. Spray with cooking spray. Add beef. Scramble-fry for about 5 minutes until beef is no longer pink.

Add ginger and garlic. Cook for about 3 minutes, stirring occasionally, until beef is browned. Remove from heat.

Add next 6 ingredients. Stir well. Transfer to small bowl. Makes about 3 1/2 cups (875 mL) filling.

Serve beef mixture on lettuce leaves. Serves 4.

1 serving: 239 Calories; 10.2 g Total Fat (4.6 g Mono, 2.1 g Poly, 2.6 g Sat); 60 mg Cholesterol; 12 g Carbohydrate; 2 g Fibre; 26 g Protein; 263 mg Sodium

CHOICES: 3 Meat & Alternatives

Creamy Couscous Parfaits

This blend of fruit, yogurt and whole grains makes for a hearty breakfast and is also good as a healthy dessert.

Skim milk	2/3 cup	150 mL
Salt, just a pinch		
Whole-wheat couscous	1/3 cup	75 mL
Can of pineapple tidbits, drained and juice reserved	14 oz.	398 mL
Coarsely chopped kiwifruit	1 cup	250 mL
Coarsely chopped strawberries	1 cup	250 mL
Reserved pineapple juice	1/4 cup	60 mL
Chopped fresh mint	2 tbsp.	30 mL
Light sour cream	1/2 cup	125 mL
Non-fat peach yogurt	1/2 cup	125 mL
Liquid honey	1 tbsp.	15 mL
Minced crystallized ginger	1 tsp.	5 mL
Grated orange zest	1/2 tsp.	2 mL

Combine milk and salt in small saucepan. Bring to a boil. Add couscous. Stir. Remove from heat. Let stand, covered, for about 5 minutes until tender. Fluff with fork. Spread on baking sheet with sides. Freeze for 5 minutes.

Meanwhile, combine next 5 ingredients in medium bowl. Let stand for 15 minutes, stirring occasionally.

Combine remaining 5 ingredients in separate medium bowl. Add chilled couscous. Stir. Spoon half of fruit mixture into 4 parfait glasses or small bowls. Spoon couscous mixture over fruit. Top with remaining fruit mixture. Makes 4 parfaits.

1 parfait: 223 Calories; 3.1 g Total Fat (trace Mono, 0.1 Poly, 1.6 g Sat); 11 mg Cholesterol; 43 g Carbohydrate; 5 g Fibre; 6 g Protein; 67 mg Sodium

CHOICES: 1/2 Grains & Starches; 1 1/2 Fruits; 1/2 Milk & Alternatives; 1/2 Fats

Pictured on page 17.

Instant Apple Cream Oatmeal

Make this deliciously satisfying oatmeal for your family any day of the week. Boil the water, stir in the oatmeal and fruit, and it will be ready to eat by the time everyone is up and dressed.

Water	3 cups	750 mL
Quick-cooking rolled oats	1/2 cup	125 mL
Quick-cooking rolled oats	1 cup	250 mL
Chopped dried apples	1/2 cup	125 mL
Skim milk powder	1/4 cup	60 mL
Brown sugar, packed	2 tbsp.	30 mL
Ground cinnamon	3/4 tsp.	4 mL
Salt	1/2 tsp.	2 mL

Bring water to a boil in medium saucepan.

Meanwhile, process first amount of oats in blender or food processor until powdery. Transfer to medium bowl.

Add remaining 6 ingredients. Stir. Slowly add to boiling water, stirring constantly. Remove from heat. Let stand, uncovered, for about 5 minutes until thickened (see Note). Makes about 3 1/2 cups (875 mL). Serves 4.

1 serving: 234 Calories; 2.3 g Total Fat (trace Mono, 0 g Poly, trace Sat); 1 mg Cholesterol; 46 g Carbohydrate; 5 g Fibre; 8 g Protein; 470 mg Sodium

CHOICES: 1 Grains & Starches; 1 Fruits; 1/2 Other Choices

Note: You can adjust the consistency of the oatmeal by adding more water.

Paré Pointer

Fast food restaurants stop thieves with a burger alarm.

Ham And Asparagus Frittata

Because frittatas are easier to make, they are sometimes thought of as shortcuts for omelets. Ham, asparagus and peppery eggs ensure there's no shortcut on flavour in this brunch favourite.

Low-cholesterol egg product	2 cups	500 mL
Grated light sharp Cheddar cheese	1/4 cup	60 mL
Skim milk	1/4 cup	60 mL
Pepper	1/2 tsp.	2 mL
Tub margarine	4 tsp.	20 mL
Chopped fresh asparagus	2 cups	500 mL
Chopped no-fat deli ham	3/4 cup	175 mL
Chopped green onion	2 tbsp.	30 mL
Grated light sharp Cheddar cheese	1/4 cup	60 mL

Preheat broiler. Whisk first 4 ingredients in medium bowl.

Melt margarine in large non-stick frying pan on medium-high. Add next 3 ingredients. Stir-fry for about 3 minutes until asparagus is tender-crisp. Pour egg mixture over asparagus mixture. Reduce heat to medium-low. Cook, covered, for about 8 minutes until almost set. Remove from heat.

Sprinkle with second amount of cheese. Broil on centre rack (see Tip, below) for about 5 minutes until cheese is melted and eggs are set. Cuts into 6 wedges.

1 wedge: 138 Calories; 6.2 g Total Fat (1.1 g Mono, 1.0 g Poly, 1.6 g Sat); 79 mg Cholesterol; 5 g Carbohydrate; 1 g Fibre; 15 g Protein; 477 mg Sodium

CHOICES: 2 Meat & Alternatives; 1/2 Fats

 tip When baking or broiling food in a frying pan with a handle that isn't ovenproof, wrap the handle in foil and keep it to the front of the oven, away from the element.

Wild Rice Apricot Pancakes

These deliciously addictive, fluffy pancakes include chewy wild rice and apricot for an interesting texture contrast. So flavourful, you could easily skip out on the butter and syrup!

Large eggs, fork-beaten	2	2
Cooked wild rice	1/2 cup	125 mL
Chopped dried apricot	1/3 cup	75 mL
Skim milk	1/3 cup	75 mL
Unsweetened applesauce	2 tbsp.	30 mL
Buttermilk pancake mix	2/3 cup	150 mL
Canola oil	2 tsp.	10 mL

Combine first 5 ingredients in small bowl. Add pancake mix. Stir until just moistened. Batter will be lumpy.

Heat 1/2 tsp. (2 mL) canola oil in large frying pan on medium. Pour batter into pan, using 1/2 cup (125 mL) for each pancake. Cook for about 2 minutes until bubbles form on top and edges appear dry. Turn pancake over. Cook for about 2 minutes until golden. Remove to plate. Cover to keep warm. Repeat with remaining batter, heating more canola oil if necessary to prevent sticking. Makes about 4 pancakes. Serves 2.

1 pancake: 198 Calories; 5.4 g Total Fat (2.7 g Mono, 1.2 g Poly, 1.0 g Sat); 93 mg Cholesterol; 31 g Carbohydrate; 2 g Fibre; 8 g Protein; 434 mg Sodium

CHOICES: 1 1/2 Grains & Starches; 1/2 Fruits; 1/2 Meat & Alternatives

Waffles With Peanut Butter Spread

Make ordinary toaster waffles extraordinary with the addition of a creamy peanut, cranberry and coconut topping.

Reduced-fat peanut butter	1/3 cup	75 mL
Light cream cheese	2 tbsp.	30 mL
Liquid honey	1 tbsp.	15 mL
Dried cranberries	2 tbsp.	30 mL
Medium unsweetened coconut	2 tbsp.	30 mL
Whole-wheat frozen waffles	8	8

Stir first 3 ingredients in small bowl until smooth.

Add cranberries and coconut. Stir. Makes about 1 cup (250 mL).

Toast waffles. Spread 2 tbsp (30 mL) peanut butter mixture over each waffle. Makes 8 waffles. Serves 4.

1 waffle: 342 Calories; 13.5 g Total Fat (1.2 g Mono, 0.6 g Poly, 4.7 g Sat); 9 mg Cholesterol; 48 g Carbohydrate; 5 g Fibre; 12 g Protein; 881 mg Sodium

CHOICES: 2 Grains & Starches; 1/2 Meat & Alternatives; 1/2 Fats

Pictured on page 17.

Chicken Salsa Wraps

The whole family will love these warm, cheesy tortillas filled with chicken and salsa. These wraps are the ultimate convenience food.

Whole-wheat flour tortillas (9 inch, 22 cm, diameter)	4	4
Salsa	1 cup	250 mL
Chopped cooked chicken (see Tip, page 38)	1 1/3 cups	325 mL
Thinly sliced red pepper	1 cup	250 mL
Grated jalapeño Monterey Jack cheese	1 cup	250 mL

(continued on next page)

Preheat oven to 400°F (205°C). Arrange tortillas on work surface. Spoon salsa down centre of each tortilla.

Layer remaining 3 ingredients over salsa. Fold bottom end of each tortilla over filling. Fold in sides. Fold over from bottom to enclose filling. Place, seam-side down, on greased baking sheet. Bake for about 15 minutes until golden. Makes 4 wraps.

1 wrap: 306 Calories; 12.1 g Total Fat (trace Mono, 1.2 g Poly, 5.0 g Sat); 64 mg Cholesterol; 26 g Carbohydrate; 4 g Fibre; 27 g Protein; 1052 mg Sodium

CHOICES: 1 Grains & Starches; 1 Vegetables; 3 Meat & Alternatives

Toasted Chicken Caesar Sandwiches

Transform your favourite meal salad into a sandwich! Makes for the perfect light lunch.

Chopped cooked chicken (see Tip, page 38)	2 cups	500 mL
Light creamy Caesar dressing	1/4 cup	60 mL
Finely chopped red onion	2 tbsp.	30 mL
Grated Romano cheese	2 tbsp.	30 mL
Real bacon bits	2 tbsp.	30 mL
Whole-wheat bread slices, toasted	4	4
Romaine lettuce leaves, torn in half	4	4
Light creamy Caesar dressing	4 tsp.	20 mL
Whole-wheat bread slices, toasted	4	4

Combine first 5 ingredients in medium bowl.

Arrange first amount of toast slices on work surface. Spread chicken mixture on toasts. Arrange lettuce over chicken mixture.

Spread second amount of Caesar dressing on remaining 4 toast slices. Place, dressing-side down, over lettuce. Press down gently. Makes 4 sandwiches.

1 sandwich: 328 Calories; 10.0 g Total Fat (3.3 g Mono, 2.1 g Poly, 2.6 g Sat); 68 mg Cholesterol; 32 g Carbohydrate; 4 g Fibre; 29 g Protein; 904 mg Sodium

CHOICES: 1 1/2 Grains & Starches; 3 Meat & Alternatives

Mango Chutney Steak Salad

Few things say summer like mango and barbecue. In this recipe, mango chutney lends its sweetness to tender grilled steak and crisp romaine. The perfect salad for a summer get-together.

Mango chutney	6 tbsp.	100 mL
Rice vinegar	3 tbsp.	50 mL
Sesame oil (for flavour)	3 tbsp.	50 mL
Soy sauce	4 tsp.	20 mL
Chili paste (sambal oelek)	3/4 tsp.	4 mL
Pepper	1/4 tsp.	1 mL
Beef strip loin steak, trimmed of fat	1 lb.	454 g
Romaine lettuce mix, lightly packed	6 cups	1.5 L
Thinly sliced yellow pepper	2 cups	500 mL

Preheat gas barbecue to medium-high. Process first 6 ingredients in blender until smooth. Transfer 1/2 cup (125 mL) chutney mixture to large bowl. Set aside.

Cook steak on greased grill for about 3 minutes per side, brushing occasionally with remaining chutney mixture, until desired doneness. Transfer to plate. Cover with foil. Let stand for 5 minutes. Cut diagonally across the grain into thin slices.

Add lettuce mix, yellow pepper and steak to reserved chutney mixture. Toss. Makes about 9 1/2 cups (2.4 L). Serves 6.

1 serving: 233 Calories; 12.8 g Total Fat (4.4 g Mono, 3.1 g Poly, 2.7 g Sat); 33 mg Cholesterol; 13 g Carbohydrate; 2 g Fibre; 18 g Protein; 382 mg Sodium

CHOICES: 1/2 Fruits; 2 Meat & Alternatives; 1 Fats

Pictured on page 35 and on back cover.

Greek Bread Salad

If croutons are your favourite part of the salad, then you must try this! Soft bread cubes absorb all the great flavour of a Dijon vinaigrette in this Greek-inspired salad.

Olive oil	1 tbsp.	15 mL
Greek seasoning	2 tsp.	10 mL
Whole-wheat bread cubes (1/2 inch, 12 mm)	3 cups	750 mL
Spring mix lettuce, lightly packed	4 cups	1 L
Chopped red pepper	1 cup	250 mL
Can of sliced black olives	1/2 cup	125 mL
Crumbled light feta cheese	1/2 cup	125 mL
Olive oil	1/3 cup	75 mL
Red wine vinegar	1/4 cup	60 mL
Dijon mustard	1 tsp.	5 mL
Dried oregano	1 tsp.	5 mL
Salt	1/2 tsp.	2 mL
Pepper	1/2 tsp.	2 mL

Preheat oven to 400°F (205°C). Combine olive oil and Greek seasoning in medium bowl. Add bread cubes. Toss until coated. Spread in single layer on ungreased baking sheet with sides. Bake for about 5 minutes, stirring at halftime, until starting to turn golden. Transfer to large bowl.

Add next 4 ingredients. Toss.

Combine remaining 6 ingredients in small cup. Drizzle over lettuce mixture. Toss. Makes about 8 cups (2 L). Serves 6.

1 serving: 242 Calories; 18.5 g Total Fat (11.8 g Mono, 1.6 g Poly, 3.6 g Sat); 7 mg Cholesterol; 15 g Carbohydrate; 3 g Fibre; 7 g Protein; 673 mg Sodium

CHOICES: 1/2 Grains & Starches; 3 Fats

Pictured on page 108.

Layered Turkey Taco Salad

With its stylish layers of delicious southwestern ingredients, this taco salad works as a super-quick weeknight supper, but it's also fancy enough for company!

Canola oil	1 tsp.	5 mL
Extra-lean ground turkey	3/4 lb.	340 g
Chili powder	2 tsp.	10 mL
Ground cumin	2 tsp.	10 mL
Salt	1/4 tsp.	1 mL
Can of black beans, rinsed and drained	19 oz.	540 mL
Frozen kernel corn	1/2 cup	125 mL
Water	1/4 cup	60 mL
Shredded iceberg lettuce, lightly packed	4 cups	1 L
Salsa	1 1/2 cups	375 mL
Light sour cream	3/4 cup	175 mL
Ripe medium avocado, diced (see Note)	1	1
Broken tortilla chips	3/4 cup	175 mL
Grated light sharp Cheddar cheese	1/2 cup	125 mL

Heat canola oil in large frying pan on medium-high. Add next 4 ingredients. Scramble-fry for about 5 minutes until no longer pink.

Add next 3 ingredients. Cook for about 5 minutes, stirring occasionally, until water is evaporated. Spread on baking sheet with sides. Cool for 5 minutes.

Put lettuce into large bowl. Spoon turkey mixture over. Layer next 5 ingredients, in order given, over turkey mixture. Makes about 10 1/2 cups (2.6 L). Serves 6.

1 serving: 300 Calories; 12.1 g Total Fat (1.0 g Mono, 0.7 g Poly, 3.2 g Sat); 38 mg Cholesterol; 30 g Carbohydrate; 7 g Fibre; 25 g Protein; 898 mg Sodium

CHOICES: 1 Grains & Starches; 3 Meat & Alternatives; 1 1/2 Fats

Note: Toss avocado with 1 tsp. (5 mL) lime juice to prevent browning.

Chorizo Bean Soup

*A classic soup gets a spicy, smoky makeover from the
addition of chorizo sausage.*

Canola oil	1 tsp.	5 mL
Chorizo sausage, casing removed	3/4 lb.	340 g
Canola oil	1 tsp.	5 mL
Chopped celery	1 cup	250 mL
Chopped onion	1 cup	250 mL
Garlic cloves, minced	2	2
(or 1/2 tsp., 2 mL, powder)		
Prepared vegetable broth	4 cups	1 L
Can of white kidney beans,	19 oz.	540 mL
rinsed and drained		
Dried rosemary, crushed	1 tsp.	5 mL
Dried thyme	1/2 tsp.	2 mL

Heat first amount of canola oil in medium frying pan on medium. Add
sausage. Scramble-fry for about 10 minutes until browned. Drain. Cover to
keep warm.

Meanwhile, heat second amount of canola oil in large saucepan on
medium-high. Add next 3 ingredients. Cook, uncovered, for about
5 minutes, stirring often, until onion is softened.

Add remaining 4 ingredients. Stir. Bring to a boil. Simmer, covered, for
10 minutes to blend flavours. Carefully process with hand blender or in
blender until smooth (see Note). Add sausage. Stir. Makes about
6 1/2 cups (1.6 L). Serves 6.

*1 serving: 218 Calories; 10.5 g Total Fat (4.4 g Mono, 1.4 g Poly, 2.9 g Sat); 16 mg Cholesterol;
20 g Carbohydrate; 5 g Fibre; 11 g Protein; 700 mg Sodium*

CHOICES: 1/2 Grains & Starches; 1 Meat & Alternatives

Note: Before processing hot liquids, check the operating instructions for
your blender.

Orange Quinoa Salad

Spicy dishes don't have to be overpowering. In this citrusy quinoa,
spicy chili paste blends perfectly with the flavours of soy, maple and orange
for a nicely warming heat.

Frozen concentrated orange juice, thawed	1/4 cup	60 mL
Rice vinegar	2 tbsp.	30 mL
Low-sodium soy sauce	1 tbsp.	15 mL
Maple (or maple-flavoured) syrup	1 tbsp.	15 mL
Chili paste (sambal oelek)	1/2 tsp.	2 mL
Garlic powder	1/2 tsp.	2 mL
Ground ginger	1/2 tsp.	2 mL
Cooked quinoa	3 cups	750 mL
Diced red pepper	1 cup	250 mL
Diced yellow pepper	1 cup	250 mL
Diced zucchini (with peel)	1 cup	250 mL

Whisk first 7 ingredients in medium bowl until combined.

Add remaining 4 ingredients. Toss. Makes about 6 cups (1.5 L). Serves 6.

1 serving: 365 Calories; 5.1 g Total Fat (1.3 g Mono, 2.1 g Poly, 0.5 g Sat); 0 mg Cholesterol;
70 g Carbohydrate; 7 g Fibre; 12 g Protein; 111 mg Sodium

CHOICES: 3 1/2 Grains & Starches

Pictured on page 35 and on back cover.

1. Shrimp And Potato Salad, page 40
2. Orange Quinoa Salad, above
3. Tropical Shrimp Fruit Salad, page 37
4. Mango Chutney Steak Salad, page 30

Props courtesy of: Cherison Enterprises Inc.

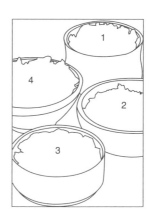

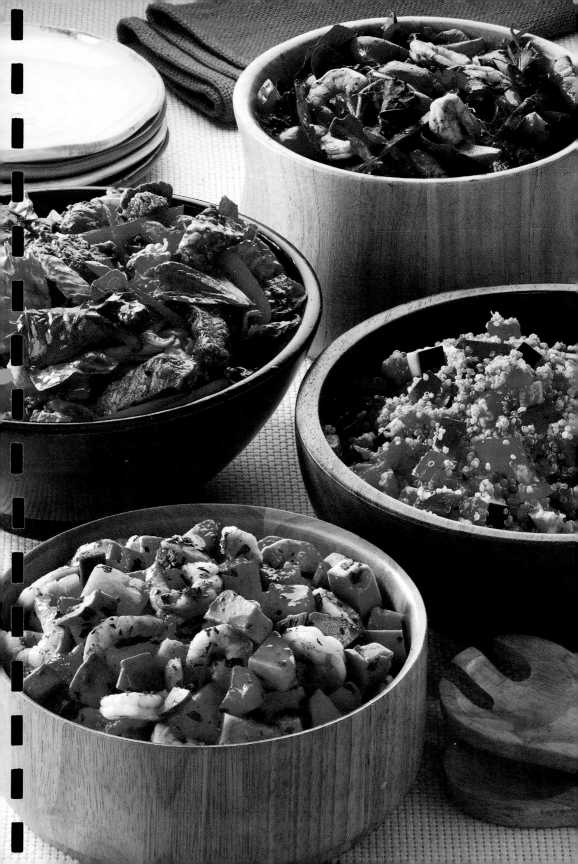

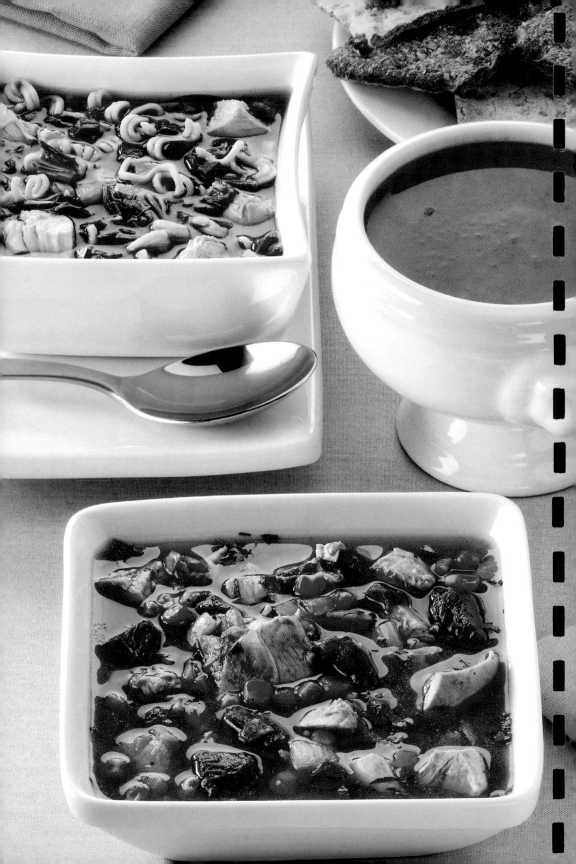

Tropical Shrimp Fruit Salad

Filled with tropical flavours, this salad is the perfect lunch for a hot summer day. Cayenne adds just a touch of heat to this refreshing combination.

Reserved pineapple juice	1/4 cup	60 mL
Chopped fresh mint	2 tbsp.	30 mL
Lime juice	2 tbsp.	30 mL
Liquid honey	2 tbsp.	30 mL
Cayenne pepper	1/4 tsp.	1 mL
Can of pineapple chunks, juice reserved	14 oz.	398 mL
Bag of frozen, cooked medium shrimp (peeled and deveined), thawed	3/4 lb.	340 g
Diced avocado	1 cup	250 mL
Frozen mango pieces, thawed and larger pieces chopped	1 cup	250 mL
Chopped celery	1/2 cup	125 mL

Combine first 5 ingredients in medium bowl.

Add remaining 5 ingredients. Toss. Let stand for 20 minutes. Makes about 6 cups (1.5 L). Serves 6.

1 serving: 184 Calories; 4.8 g Total Fat (2.6 g Mono, 0.9 g Poly, 0.8 g Sat); 86 mg Cholesterol; 24 g Carbohydrate; 3 g Fibre; 13 g Protein; 95 mg Sodium

CHOICES: 1 Fruits; 1/2 Other Choices; 1 1/2 Meat & Alternatives; 1 Fats

Pictured on page 35 and on back cover.

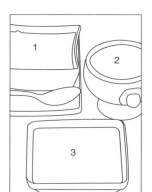

1. Five-Spice Chicken Noodle Soup, page 38
2. Pumpkin Apple Soup, page 44
3. Chicken Corn Soup, page 41

Props courtesy of: Danesco Inc.
Cherison Enterprises Inc.
Casa Bugatti

Soups & Salads

Five-Spice Chicken Noodle Soup

Asian flavours are just a few minutes away when you cook this fabulous soup in your microwave. Just as fast as packaged instant noodles, but a whole lot tastier!

Low-sodium prepared chicken broth	4 cups	1 L
Low-sodium soy sauce	1 tbsp.	15 mL
Chinese five-spice powder	1/4 tsp.	1 mL
Garlic powder	1/4 tsp.	1 mL
Ground ginger	1/8 tsp.	0.5 mL
Chopped bok choy	2 cups	500 mL
Dry, thin Chinese-style instant noodles, broken up	3.25 oz.	100 g
Finely chopped red pepper	1/4 cup	60 mL
Sliced green onion	2 tbsp.	30 mL
Chopped cooked chicken (see Tip, below)	1 1/2 cups	375 mL

Combine first 5 ingredients in large microwave-safe bowl. Microwave, covered, on high (100%) for about 10 minutes until boiling.

Add next 4 ingredients. Stir. Microwave, covered, on high (100%) for about 2 minutes until noodles are tender.

Add chicken. Stir. Microwave, uncovered, on high (100%) for about 1 minute until heated through. Makes about 6 1/2 cups (1.6 L). Serves 4.

1 serving: 213 Calories; 5.3 g Total Fat (1.5 g Mono, 1.0 g Poly, 1.2 g Sat); 67 mg Cholesterol; 14 g Carbohydrate; 1 g Fibre; 26 g Protein; 1040 mg Sodium

CHOICES: 1/2 Grains & Starches; 2 Meat & Alternatives

Pictured on page 36.

 Don't have any leftover chicken? Start with 2 boneless, skinless chicken breast halves (4 – 6 oz., 113 – 170 g, each). Place in large frying pan with 1 cup (250 mL) water or chicken broth. Simmer, covered, for 12 to 14 minutes until no longer pink inside. Drain. Chop. Makes about 2 cups (500 mL) of cooked chicken.

Fennel And Grapefruit Soup

Ready to try something completely new? Caramelizing onion and fennel brings out a natural sweetness that is brightened by tart grapefruit juice. These flavours go surprisingly well together!

Canola oil	2 tsp.	10 mL
Chopped fennel bulb (white part only)	2 cups	500 mL
Chopped onion	1/2 cup	125 mL
Garlic clove, minced	1	1
(or 1/4 tsp., 1 mL, powder)		
Fennel seeds	1/2 tsp.	2 mL
Ground ginger	1/4 tsp.	1 mL
Brown sugar, packed	1 tsp.	5 mL
Low-sodium prepared chicken broth	2 cups	500 mL
Red grapefruit juice	1/4 cup	60 mL
Instant potato flakes	1/2 cup	125 mL
2% evaporated milk	1/2 cup	125 mL

Sliced green onion, for garnish

Heat canola oil in large saucepan on medium. Add next 5 ingredients. Cook for about 10 minutes, stirring often, until fennel and onion start to brown.

Add sugar. Heat and stir for about 1 minute until fennel and onion are golden.

Add broth and juice. Stir. Bring to a boil. Add potato flakes. Heat and stir until boiling and thickened. Add evaporated milk. Cook and stir until heated through. Carefully process with hand blender or in blender until smooth (see Note).

Garnish with green onion. Makes about 4 cups (1 L). Serves 4.

1 serving: 158 Calories; 3.4 g Total Fat (1.6 g Mono, 0.7 g Poly, 0.6 g Sat); 5 mg Cholesterol; 28 g Carbohydrate; 7 g Fibre; 7 g Protein; 441 mg Sodium

CHOICES: 2 Vegetables; 1/2 Fats

Note: Before processing hot liquids, check the operating instructions for your blender.

Shrimp And Potato Salad

Get your protein, carbs and greens—all together in a tasty salad! Shrimp, potatoes and crisp, fresh veggies mingle in a balsamic and Dijon vinaigrette.

Baby potatoes, quartered	1 lb.	454 g
Water	1/4 cup	60 mL
Montreal steak spice	1/2 tsp.	2 mL
Balsamic vinegar	2 tbsp.	30 mL
Olive (or canola) oil	2 tbsp.	30 mL
Dijon mustard	2 tsp.	10 mL
Salt	1/4 tsp.	1 mL
Pepper	1/4 tsp.	1 mL
Spring mix lettuce, lightly packed	4 cups	1 L
Cooked medium shrimp	1/2 lb.	225 g
(peeled and deveined)		
Thinly sliced red pepper	1/2 cup	125 mL

Put potato and water into medium microwave-safe bowl. Microwave, covered, on high (100%) for about 10 minutes, stirring every 3 minutes, until tender. Rinse with cold water. Drain. Add steak spice. Toss.

Meanwhile, combine next 5 ingredients in large bowl. Makes about 1/3 cup (75 mL) dressing.

Add remaining 3 ingredients and potato. Toss. Makes about 8 cups (2 L). Serves 8.

1 cup (250 mL): 117 Calories; 3.9 g Total Fat (2.6 g Mono, 0.5 g Poly, 0.6 g Sat); 43 mg Cholesterol; 12 g Carbohydrate; 1 g Fibre; 8 g Protein; 177 mg Sodium

CHOICES: 1/2 Grains & Starches; 1 Meat & Alternatives; 1/2 Fats

Pictured on page 35.

 Chipotle chili peppers are smoked jalapeño peppers. Be sure to wash your hands after handling. To store any leftover chipotle chili peppers, divide into recipe-friendly portions and freeze, with sauce, in airtight containers for up to one year.

Chicken Corn Soup

*Your standard chicken soup just went south of the border and
came back loaded with exciting new flavours.*

Canola oil	1 tsp.	5 mL
Frozen kernel corn	2 cups	500 mL
Chopped onion	1 cup	250 mL
Garlic cloves, minced	2	2
(or 1/2 tsp., 2 mL, powder)		
Finely chopped chipotle pepper in	1/2 tsp.	2 mL
adobo sauce (see Tip, page 40)		
Low-sodium prepared chicken broth	3 cups	750 mL
Can of diced tomatoes (with juice)	14 oz.	398 mL
Pepper	1/4 tsp.	1 mL
Chopped cooked chicken	2 cups	500 mL
(see Tip, page 38)		
Chopped fresh cilantro	1 tbsp.	15 mL
Lime juice	1 tbsp.	15 mL

Heat canola oil in large saucepan on medium-high. Add next 4 ingredients.
Cook, uncovered, for about 4 minutes, stirring often, until onion is softened.

Add next 3 ingredients. Stir. Bring to a boil. Reduce heat to medium. Boil
gently, covered, for 6 minutes to blend flavours.

Add chicken. Cook and stir for about 3 minutes until heated through.

Add cilantro and lime juice. Stir. Makes about 7 cups (1.75 L). Serves 6.

*1 serving: 201 Calories; 5.6 g Total Fat (1.8 g Mono, 1.1 g Poly, 1.1 g Sat); 58 mg Cholesterol;
16 g Carbohydrate; 1 g Fibre; 22 g Protein; 699 mg Sodium*

CHOICES: 1/2 Grains & Starches; 1/2 Vegetables; 1 1/2 Meat &
Alternatives

Pictured on page 36.

Bean Medley Soup

A hearty meatless soup with the spicy flavour of chipotle pepper and the freshness of lime. Adding a garnish of sour cream and cilantro will give this flavourful soup a little extra punch.

Olive (or canola) oil	2 tsp.	10 mL
Chopped onion	1 cup	250 mL
Garlic cloves, minced	2	2
(or 1/2 tsp., 2 mL, powder)		
Ground cumin	1 tsp.	5 mL
Prepared vegetable broth	3 cups	750 mL
Can of mixed beans, rinsed and drained	19 oz.	540 mL
Can of navy beans, rinsed and drained	14 oz.	398 mL
Finely chopped chipotle peppers	2 tsp.	10 mL
in adobo sauce (see Tip, page 40)		
Lime juice	1 tbsp.	15 mL

Heat olive oil in large saucepan on medium. Add next 3 ingredients. Cook, uncovered, for about 5 minutes, stirring often, until onion is softened.

Add next 4 ingredients. Bring to a boil. Reduce heat to medium-low. Simmer, partially covered, for 10 minutes, stirring occasionally. Remove 1 cup (250 mL) of solids. Mash. Add to soup. Stir.

Add lime juice. Stir. Makes about 6 cups (1.5 L). Serves 4.

1 serving: 282 Calories; 3.8 g Total Fat (1.7 g Mono, 0.4 g Poly, 0.4 g Sat); 0 mg Cholesterol; 49 g Carbohydrate; 12 g Fibre; 16 g Protein; 958 mg Sodium

CHOICES: 2 Grains & Starches; 2 Meat & Alternatives; 1/2 Fats

Tuna Chowder

This chowder gets its thick and hearty texture from grated potato instead of rich milk or cream—what a concept!

Prepared vegetable broth	4 cups	1 L
Frozen cut green beans	2 cups	500 mL
Grated peeled potato	2 cups	500 mL
Dried basil	1/2 tsp.	2 mL
Dried thyme	1/4 tsp.	1 mL
Pepper	1/4 tsp.	1 mL
Olive oil	1 tsp.	5 mL
Chopped onion	1 cup	250 mL
Chopped green pepper	1/2 cup	125 mL
Garlic clove, minced	1	1
(or 1/4 tsp., 1 mL, powder)		
Can of chunk light tuna in water, drained	6 oz.	170 g

Bring broth to a boil in large saucepan. Add next 5 ingredients. Reduce heat to medium. Boil gently, covered, for 10 minutes, stirring occasionally.

Heat olive oil in small frying pan on medium. Add next 3 ingredients. Cook for about 5 minutes, stirring often, until onion is softened. Add to broth mixture.

Add tuna. Stir. Simmer, covered, for about 2 minutes until heated through. Makes about 7 1/2 cups (1.9 L). Serves 6.

1 serving: 130 Calories; 5 g Total Fat (2.0 g Mono, 0.6 g Poly, 1.4 g Sat); 9 mg Cholesterol; 19 g Carbohydrate; 3 g Fibre; 10 g Protein; 339 mg Sodium

CHOICES: 1/2 Grains & Starches; 1 Vegetables; 1 Meat & Alternatives

Pumpkin Apple Soup

Harvest from your pantry for the ingredients to make this light and delicious soup. It's easy enough for a quick lunch, sophisticated enough for a dinner party and easily doubled so you'll have lots left over.

Prepared chicken broth	2 cups	500 mL
Can of pure pumpkin (no spices)	14 oz.	398 mL
Unsweetened applesauce	1 cup	250 mL
Ground cinnamon	1/2 tsp.	2 mL
Ground cumin	1/4 tsp.	1 mL
Skim evaporated milk	1/2 cup	125 mL

Combine first 5 ingredients in medium saucepan. Bring to a boil, stirring occasionally.

Add evaporated milk. Heat and stir for 1 minute. Makes about 5 cups (1.25 L). Serves 4.

1 serving: 97 Calories; 1.0 g Total Fat (0.3 g Mono, 0.2 g Poly, 0.3 g Sat); 1 mg Cholesterol; 20 g Carbohydrate; 4 g Fibre; 4 g Protein; 785 mg Sodium

CHOICES: 1/2 Fruits; 1 Vegetables

Pictured on page 36.

Curly Ribbon Salad

Like presents, some meals are best when topped with ribbons! Serve this pretty salad and see for yourself.

Chopped fresh basil	3 tbsp.	50 mL
White vinegar	2 tbsp.	30 mL
Olive oil	1 tbsp.	15 mL
Granulated sugar	2 tsp.	10 mL
Salt	1/4 tsp.	1 mL
Thinly sliced English cucumber (with peel), see Note	3 cups	750 mL
Thinly sliced peeled daikon radish (see Note)	2 cups	500 mL

(continued on next page)

44 Soups & Salads

Whisk first 5 ingredients in large bowl until sugar is dissolved.

Add cucumber and daikon. Toss until coated. Makes about 3 1/2 cups (875 mL). Serves 4.

1 serving: 65 Calories; 4.5 g Total Fat (2.5 g Mono, 0.3 g Poly, 0.5 g Sat); 0 mg Cholesterol; 6 g Carbohydrate; trace Fibre; 2 g Protein; 148 mg Sodium

CHOICES: 1/2 Fats

Note: Use a vegetable peeler to cut long, thin, ribbon-like slices.

Chard And Hazelnut Salad

Sweet mandarin orange, salty blue cheese and toasted hazelnuts combine in a deep green salad—the flavours intermingle in the most delightful way!

Chopped or torn ruby (or Swiss) chard, lightly packed	4 cups	1 L
Can of mandarin orange segments, drained and juice reserved	10 oz.	284 mL
Coarsely chopped hazelnuts (filberts), toasted (see Tip, page 114)	1/2 cup	125 mL
Thinly sliced red onion	1/2 cup	125 mL
Crumbled blue cheese	1/4 cup	60 mL
ORANGE DRESSING		
Olive (or canola) oil	3 tbsp.	50 mL
Red wine vinegar	2 tbsp.	30 mL
Reserved mandarin orange juice	2 tbsp.	30 mL
Granulated sugar	1 tbsp.	15 mL
Salt	1/4 tsp.	1 mL

Combine first 5 ingredients in large bowl.

Orange Dressing: Combine all 5 ingredients in jar with tight-fitting lid. Shake well. Makes about 1/2 cup (125 mL) dressing. Drizzle over salad. Toss. Makes about 6 cups (1.5 L). Serves 4.

1 serving: 258 Calories; 21.0 g Total Fat (14.0 g Mono, 2.0 g Poly, 3.3 g Sat); 6 mg Cholesterol; 16 g Carbohydrate; 3 g Fibre; 5 g Protein; 322 mg Sodium

CHOICES: 1/2 Fruits; 4 Fats

White Bean Hummus And Pita Chips

A hearty helping of hummus and pita makes for an unbeatable snack. This version uses white beans and replaces the tahini with lower-fat yogurt and sesame oil. Baked whole-wheat pita chips make the perfect dipper.

WHITE BEAN HUMMUS

Can of white kidney beans, rinsed and drained	19 oz.	540 mL
Lemon juice	2 tbsp.	30 mL
Low-fat plain yogurt	1/3 cup	75 mL
Sesame oil (for flavour)	2 tsp.	10 mL
Garlic clove, minced (or 1/4 tsp., 1 mL, powder)	1	1
Ground cumin	1/2 tsp.	2 mL
Salt	1/4 tsp.	1 mL
Pepper	1/4 tsp.	1 mL

PITA CHIPS

Whole-wheat pita breads (7 inch, 18 cm, diameter)	4	4
Cooking spray		
Salt, sprinkle		
Pepper, sprinkle		

White Bean Hummus: Preheat oven to 375°F (190°C). Process all 8 ingredients in blender or food processor until smooth. Makes about 1 1/2 cups (375 mL) hummus.

Pita Chips: Spray 1 side of each pita bread with cooking spray. Sprinkle with salt and pepper. Stack pitas. Cut stack into 8 wedges. Spread in single layer on ungreased baking sheet. Bake for about 10 minutes until crisp and golden. Serve with hummus. Makes 32 pita chips.

1/4 cup (60 mL) hummus with 5 pita chips: 207 Calories; 3.5 g Total Fat (0.7 g Mono, 1.1 g Poly, 0.5 g Sat); 1 mg Cholesterol; 37 g Carbohydrate; 7 g Fibre; 9 g Protein; 362 mg Sodium

CHOICES: 2 Grains & Starches; 1/2 Meat & Alternatives

Chocolate Chip Softies

Like a white lie—using mini-chips makes it look like there's more chocolate in these satisfying bite-sized cookies. Everyone is sure to enjoy these soft little cookies, and applesauce replaces some of the butter and sugar.

Tub margarine	1/4 cup	60 mL
Granulated sugar	1/4 cup	60 mL
Unsweetened applesauce	1/4 cup	60 mL
Skim milk	1 tbsp.	15 mL
Egg white	1	1
Vanilla extract	1 tsp.	5 mL
All-purpose flour	3/4 cup	175 mL
Mini semi-sweet chocolate chips	1/4 cup	60 mL
Baking soda	1/4 tsp.	1 mL
Salt	1/8 tsp.	0.5 mL

Preheat oven to 375°F (190°C). Cream margarine and sugar in medium bowl until fluffy. Beat in next 4 ingredients.

Add remaining 4 ingredients. Stir. Drop, using about 1 tbsp. (15 mL) for each, about 1 inch (2.5 cm) apart onto greased cookie sheet. Bake for about 10 minutes until golden. Let stand on cookie sheet for 5 minutes. Remove cookies from cookie sheet and place on wire rack to cool. Makes about 16 cookies.

1 cookie: 77 Calories; 3.9 g Total Fat (1.5 g Mono, 1.2 g Poly, 1.0 g Sat); trace Cholesterol; 10 g Carbohydrate; trace Fibre; 1 g Protein; 80 mg Sodium

CHOICES: 1/2 Other Choices; 1/2 Fats

Pictured on page 144.

Paré Pointer

If you sell mobile homes, are you a wheel estate agent?

Banana Oat Muffins

These bite-sized muffins are loaded with the goodness of oats, banana, peanut butter and whole wheat for a satisfying snack—you may just forget that they're good for you! Processing the wet ingredients ensures even distribution throughout the muffins.

Large flake rolled oats	1 cup	250 mL
All-purpose flour	1/2 cup	125 mL
Whole-wheat flour	1/2 cup	125 mL
Brown sugar, packed	1/4 cup	60 mL
Baking powder	1 tbsp.	15 mL
Ground cinnamon	1 tsp.	5 mL
Ground cardamom	1/2 tsp.	2 mL
Salt	1/4 tsp.	1 mL
Large egg	1	1
Overripe medium banana (see Tip, below)	1	1
Milk	1/2 cup	125 mL
Peanut butter	1/3 cup	75 mL
Vanilla extract	1 tsp.	5 mL

Preheat oven to 375°F (190°C). Measure first 8 ingredients into large mixing bowl. Make a well in centre.

Process remaining 5 ingredients in blender or food processor until smooth. Add to well. Stir until just moistened. Fill 24 greased mini-muffin cups. Bake for about 12 minutes until lightly browned and wooden pick inserted in centre of muffin comes out clean. Let stand in pan for 5 minutes. Remove muffins from pan and place on wire rack to cool. Makes 24 mini-muffins.

1 mini-muffin: 71 Calories; 2.4 g Total Fat (1.0 g Mono, 0.6 g Poly, 0.5 g Sat); 8 mg Cholesterol; 11 g Carbohydrate; 1 g Fibre; 3 g Protein; 64 mg Sodium

CHOICES: 1/2 Grains & Starches

 tip When your bananas get too ripe to enjoy fresh, peel and cut them into 2 inch (5 cm) chunks and freeze on a baking sheet. Once frozen, transfer to freezer bag for use in any blended beverage. Ripe bananas have superior flavour for beverages.

Berry Minty Smoothie

Fresh mint adds a refreshing coolness to this creamy blend of berries and bananas. If you don't like the seeds in blackberries, choose a berry mix without them or just pick the blackberries out before measuring.

Frozen mixed berries	1 1/2 cups	375 mL
Overripe medium banana, cut up (see Tip, page 48)	1	1
Soy milk	1/2 cup	125 mL
Ground flaxseed	1 tbsp.	15 mL
Fresh mint leaves	6	6

Process all 5 ingredients in blender or food processor until smooth. Makes about 1 3/4 cups (425 mL). Serves 2.

1 serving: 152 Calories; 1.9 g Total Fat (0.3 g Mono, 0.5 g Poly, 0.2 g Sat); 0 mg Cholesterol; 31 g Carbohydrate; 7 g Fibre; 5 g Protein; 34 mg Sodium

CHOICES: 1 1/2 Fruits

Peppered Popcorn

Transform ordinary microwave popcorn into a peppery, flavourful treat with the addition of a spicy secret ingredient.

Tub margarine	2 tbsp.	30 mL
Cayenne pepper	1/2 tsp.	2 mL
Bag of trans fat-free microwave popcorn	3 oz.	85 g

Combine margarine and cayenne pepper in small microwave-safe bowl. Microwave, uncovered, on high (100%) for about 30 seconds until margarine is melted. Stir.

Microwave popcorn on high (100%) for 2 to 3 minutes until popping slows to 1 second between pops. Carefully remove bag from microwave. Transfer popcorn to extra-large bowl. Drizzle with margarine mixture. Toss until coated. Makes about 11 cups (2.75 L).

1 cup (250 mL): 52 Calories; 2.8 g Total Fat (1.2 g Mono, 1.1 g Poly, 0.4 g Sat); 0 mg Cholesterol; 6 g Carbohydrate; 1 g Fibre; 1 g Protein; 66 mg Sodium

CHOICES: 1/2 Fats

Razzle-Dazzle Smoothie

The addition of chocolate makes this raspberry smoothie dazzle! Forget fat-filled milkshakes—this nutritious beverage is the best way to get your next chocolate fix.

Frozen whole raspberries	2 cups	500 mL
Non-fat raspberry yogurt	2 cups	500 mL
Light hot chocolate mix	1/2 cup	125 mL
Skim milk	1/2 cup	125 mL
Large banana, sliced	1	1
Ice cubes	8	8

Process all 6 ingredients in blender or food processor until smooth. Makes about 5 cups (1.25 L). Serves 4.

1 serving: 230 Calories; 0.7 g Total Fat (trace Mono, trace Poly, 0.1 g Sat); 3 mg Cholesterol; 43 g Carbohydrate; 7 g Fibre; 13 g Protein; 534 mg Sodium

CHOICES: 2 1/2 Fruits; 1 Milk & Alternatives

Pictured on page 54.

Blueberry Smoothie

Double the flavours, double the taste! A double-dose of blueberry flavour is rounded out by milk and vanilla for a quick and satisfying snack.

Frozen blueberries	1 1/2 cups	375 mL
Non-fat blueberry yogurt	1 cup	250 mL
Skim milk	3/4 cup	175 mL
Skim milk powder	2 tbsp.	30 mL
Vanilla extract	1 tsp.	5 mL

Process all 5 ingredients in blender or food processor until smooth. Makes about 3 cups (750 mL). Serves 2.

1 serving: 183 Calories; 1.0 g Total Fat (0.1 g Mono, trace Poly, 0.1 g Sat); 6 mg Cholesterol; 33 g Carbohydrate; 3 g Fibre; 11 g Protein; 145 mg Sodium

CHOICES: 1/2 Fruits; 1 1/2 Milk & Alternatives

Pictured on page 54.

Pumpkin Power Puffs

These fibre and protein-packed puffs are a cross between a muffin and a cookie, each topped with a big chocolate kiss!

All-purpose flour	3/4 cup	175 mL
Whole-wheat flour	3/4 cup	175 mL
Brown sugar, packed	1/2 cup	125 mL
Baking powder	1 1/2 tsp.	7 mL
Ground cinnamon	1/2 tsp.	2 mL
Salt	1/4 tsp.	1 mL
Ground nutmeg	1/8 tsp.	0.5 mL
Ground cloves, just a pinch		
Large egg	1	1
Canned navy beans, rinsed and drained	1/2 cup	125 mL
Canned pure pumpkin (no spices)	1/2 cup	125 mL
Milk	3 tbsp.	50 mL
Canola oil	2 tbsp.	30 mL
Vanilla extract	1 tsp.	5 mL
Chocolate rosette candies	27	27

Preheat oven to 375°F (190°C). Combine first 8 ingredients in large bowl. Make a well in centre.

Process next 6 ingredients in blender or food processor until smooth. Add to well. Stir until just moistened. Drop, using 1 tbsp. (15 mL) for each, about 1 inch (2.5 cm) apart onto 2 greased cookie sheets (see Note).

Press one chocolate rosette, pointed-side down, into centre of each cookie. Bake on separate racks in oven for about 12 minutes, switching position of cookie sheets at halftime, until bottoms are golden. Let stand on cookie sheets for 5 minutes. Remove cookies from cookie sheets and place on wire racks to cool. Makes about 27 puffs.

1 puff: 84 Calories; 2.8 g Total Fat (0.7 g Mono, 0.4 g Poly, 1.1 g Sat); 8 mg Cholesterol; 13 g Carbohydrate; 1 g Fibre; 2 g Protein; 63 mg Sodium

CHOICES: 1/2 Other Choices

Pictured on page 144.

Note: To save time, use a small self-clearing ice cream scoop to portion the cookies easily and uniformly.

Cocoa Coconut Macaroons

It's unlikely that there's a more fitting combination than chocolate and coconut. These light cookies are quick to make and so good that they'll probably disappear just as fast.

Box of angel food cake mix	15 oz.	430 g
Medium unsweetened coconut	1 cup	250 mL
Cocoa, sifted if lumpy	1/4 cup	60 mL
Water	1/3 cup	75 mL

Preheat oven to 300°F (150°C). Combine first 3 ingredients in medium bowl.

Add water. Mix well. Drop, using about 1 tbsp. (15 mL) for each, about 2 inches (5 cm) apart onto 2 greased cookie sheets. Flatten with fork. Bake on separate racks in oven for about 12 minutes, switching position of cookie sheets at halftime, until cookies are crisp. Let stand on cookie sheets for 5 minutes. Remove cookies from cookie sheets and place on wire racks to cool. Makes about 40 cookies.

1 cookie: 53 Calories; 1.3 g Total Fat (0.1 g Mono, trace Poly, 1.1 g Sat); 0 mg Cholesterol; 10 g Carbohydrate; trace Fibre; 1 g Protein; 79 mg Sodium

CHOICES: 1/2 Other Choices

Pictured on page 144.

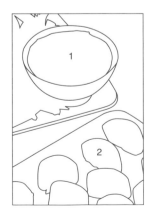

1. Thai Spinach Dip, page 58
2. Veggie Pinwheels, page 60

Props courtesy of: Danesco Inc.

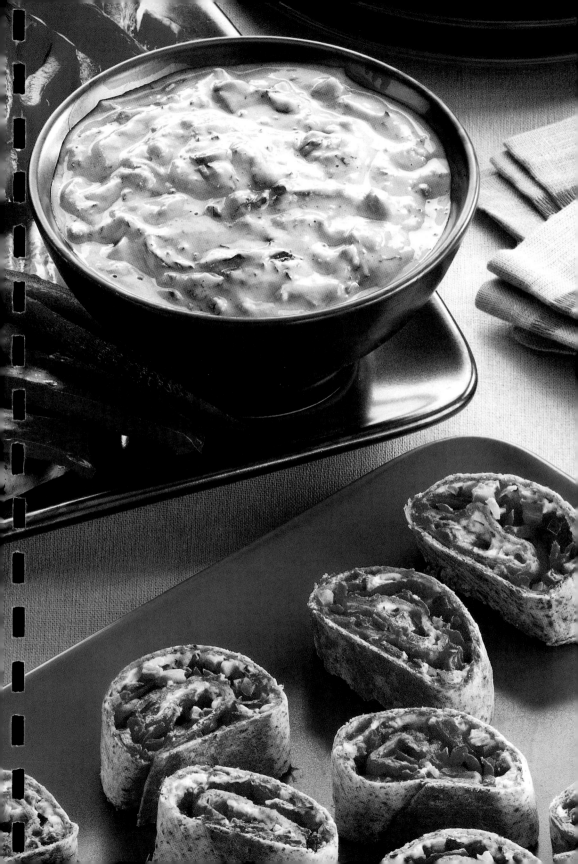

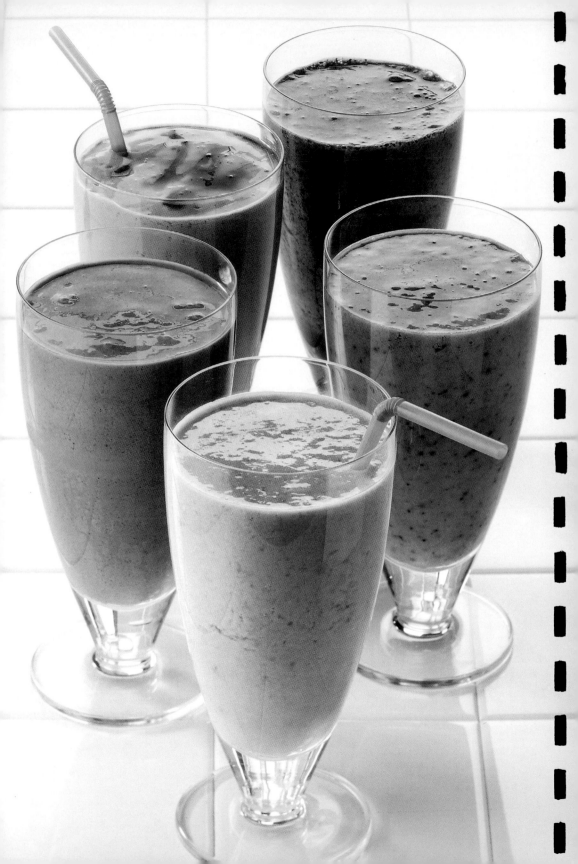

Peppermint Patty Puffs

These dense, brownie-like cupcakes pack some peppermint punch! Just as satisfying as the ever-popular mint and chocolate treat they're named for.

Semi-sweet chocolate baking squares (1 oz., 28 g, each), chopped	2	2
Granulated sugar	1 cup	250 mL
All-purpose flour	1/2 cup	125 mL
Cocoa, sifted if lumpy	1/2 cup	125 mL
Salt	1/4 tsp.	1 mL
Large eggs, fork-beaten	2	2
Unsweetened applesauce	1/2 cup	125 mL
Peppermint extract	1/2 tsp.	2 mL

Preheat oven to 350°F (175°C). Put chocolate into small microwave-safe bowl. Microwave on medium (50%) for about 90 seconds, stirring every 30 seconds, until almost melted. Stir until smooth.

Combine next 4 ingredients in medium bowl. Make a well in centre.

Whisk remaining 3 ingredients and melted chocolate in small bowl. Add to well. Stir until just moistened. Fill 24 greased mini-muffin cups 3/4 full. Bake for 12 to 15 minutes until wooden pick inserted in centre of puff comes out clean. Do not overbake. Makes 24 puffs.

1 puff: 62 Calories; 1.0 g Total Fat (0.4 g Mono, 0.1 g Poly, 0.5 g Sat); 16 mg Cholesterol; 13 g Carbohydrate; 1 g Fibre; 1 g Protein; 30 mg Sodium

CHOICES: 1/2 Other Choices

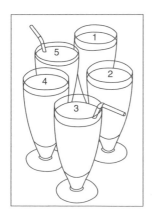

1. Blueberry Smoothie, page 50
2. Razzle-Dazzle Smoothie, page 50
3. Tropical Tango Tofu Smoothie, page 60
4. Tart Cranberry Refresher, page 58
5. Caramel Mocha Smoothie, page 61

Props courtesy of: The Bay

Chocolate Crackle Cakes

With portion sizes just large enough for a tiny treat, even white chocolate can be part of a healthy diet. We've used just enough to suggest decadence, but these crackle cakes won't send your blood sugar skyrocketing.

Large egg	1	1
Granulated sugar	1/3 cup	75 mL
Canola oil	2 tbsp.	30 mL
Vanilla extract	1 1/2 tsp.	7 mL
All-purpose flour	2/3 cup	150 mL
Baking powder	1/4 tsp.	1 mL
Salt	1/8 tsp.	0.5 mL
White chocolate baking square (1 oz., 28 g), chopped	1	1

Preheat oven to 350°F (175°C). Whisk first 4 ingredients in medium bowl until smooth.

Add next 3 ingredients. Whisk until combined.

Put chocolate into small microwave-safe bowl. Microwave, uncovered, on medium (50%) for about 45 seconds, stirring every 15 seconds, until chocolate is almost melted. Stir until smooth. Add to batter. Fill 12 greased mini-muffin cups 3/4 full. Bake for 10 to 12 minutes until wooden pick inserted in centre of cake comes out clean. Let stand in pan for 5 minutes. Remove cakes from pan and place on wire rack to cool. Makes 12 cakes.

1 cake: 83 Calories; 4.0 g Total Fat (2.0 g Mono, 0.8 g Poly, 1.1 g Sat); 16 mg Cholesterol; 11 g Carbohydrate; trace Fibre; 1 g Protein; 35 mg Sodium

CHOICES: 1/2 Fats; 1/2 Other Choices

Paré Pointer

Guess who fell down the chimney last Christmas? Santa Klutz.

Chocolate Orange Muffins

There's a secret ingredient in these muffins, and no one will ever guess what it is. Beans add lots of fibre and protein while a shiny orange glaze gives the appearance of party fare.

All-purpose flour	1 1/4 cups	300 mL
Whole-wheat flour	3/4 cup	175 mL
Cocoa, sifted if lumpy	1/4 cup	60 mL
Baking powder	2 tsp.	10 mL
Salt	1/2 tsp.	2 mL
Large eggs	2	2
Canned white kidney beans, rinsed and drained	1 cup	250 mL
Skim milk	2/3 cup	150 mL
Brown sugar, packed	1/2 cup	125 mL
Canola oil	1/4 cup	60 mL
Frozen concentrated orange juice, thawed	2 tbsp.	30 mL
Brown sugar, packed	1 tbsp.	15 mL

Preheat oven to 400°F (205°C). Measure first 5 ingredients into large bowl. Stir. Make a well in centre.

Process next 5 ingredients in blender or food processor until smooth. Add to well. Stir until just moistened. Fill 12 greased muffin cups 2/3 full. Bake for about 15 minutes until wooden pick inserted in centre of muffin comes out clean.

Meanwhile, combine concentrated orange juice and second amount of sugar in small cup. Brush over tops of hot muffins. Let stand in pan for 5 minutes. Remove muffins from pan and place on wire rack to cool. Makes 12 muffins.

1 muffin: 189 Calories; 5.9 g Total Fat (3.1 g Mono, 1.5 g Poly, 0.8 g Sat); 31 mg Cholesterol; 30 g Carbohydrate; 2 g Fibre; 5 g Protein; 169 mg Sodium

CHOICES: 1 Grains & Starches; 1/2 Other Choices; 1 Fats

Thai Spinach Dip

The fresh, light flavours of Thai cuisine shine in a rich and creamy spinach dip. Dunk in your favourite cut-up vegetables and enjoy!

Olive (or canola) oil	1 tsp.	5 mL
Chopped onion	1/2 cup	125 mL
Dried crushed chilies	1/2 tsp.	2 mL
Chopped fresh spinach leaves, lightly packed	1 cup	250 mL
Light sour cream	1/2 cup	125 mL
Non-fat plain yogurt	1/2 cup	125 mL
Light chunky peanut butter	3 tbsp.	50 mL
Chopped fresh mint	2 tbsp.	30 mL
Lime juice	1 tbsp.	15 mL
Liquid honey	1 tbsp.	15 mL
Low-sodium soy sauce	1 1/2 tsp.	7 mL

Heat olive oil in small frying pan on medium. Add onion and chilies. Cook for about 5 minutes, stirring often, until onion is softened.

Add spinach. Heat and stir for about 1 minute until wilted. Remove from heat.

Whisk remaining 7 ingredients in medium bowl. Add spinach mixture. Stir. Makes about 1 1/2 cups (375 mL).

3 tbsp. (50 mL): 85 Calories; 4.3 g Total Fat (0.4 g Mono, trace Poly, 1.5 g Sat); 6 mg Cholesterol; 8 g Carbohydrate; 1 Fibre; 3 g Protein; 96 mg Sodium

CHOICES: 1/2 Fats

Pictured on page 53.

Tart Cranberry Refresher

You'll be tickled pink by the tart flavours of cranberry and raspberry in this refreshing pink smoothie.

Non-fat raspberry yogurt	2 cups	500 mL
Frozen raspberries	1 cup	250 mL
Cranberry juice	1/2 cup	125 mL
Frozen cranberries	1/2 cup	125 mL

(continued on next page)

Process all 4 ingredients in blender or food processor until smooth. Makes about 3 1/2 cups (875 mL). Serves 2.

1 serving: 211 Calories; 0.6 g Total Fat (0 g Mono, 0 g Poly, 0 g Sat); 5 mg Cholesterol; 44 g Carbohydrate; 4 g Fibre; 9 g Protein; 117 mg Sodium

CHOICES: 1 Fruits; 1 1/2 Milk & Alternatives

Pictured on page 54.

Quick PB Cookies

If you love peanut butter cookies, you can feel free to indulge in this healthier version. Light peanut butter and applesauce provide most of the sweetness and help to reduce the fat.

Large egg, fork-beaten	1	1
Chunky light peanut butter	1 cup	250 mL
Unsweetened applesauce	1/4 cup	60 mL
Granulated sugar	3 tbsp.	50 mL
All-purpose flour	1/4 cup	60 mL
Baking powder	1/4 tsp.	1 mL

Preheat oven to 325°F (160°C). Combine first 4 ingredients in medium bowl.

Add flour and baking powder. Mix until no white streaks remain. Drop, using about 1 tbsp. (15 mL) for each, about 2 inches (5 cm) apart onto 2 ungreased cookie sheets. Bake on separate racks in oven for about 12 minutes, switching position of cookie sheets at halftime, until edges are golden. Let stand on cookie sheets for 5 minutes. Remove cookies from cookie sheets and place on wire racks to cool. Makes about 21 cookies.

1 cookie: 89 Calories; 4.8 g Total Fat (0.1 g Mono, trace Poly, 1.0 g Sat); 9 mg Cholesterol; 9 g Carbohydrate; 1 g Fibre; 3 g Protein; 90 mg Sodium

CHOICES: 1/2 Meat & Alternatives

Pictured on page 144.

Tropical Tango Tofu Smoothie

You may not think of healthy drinks as being rich, creamy and sweet—but this sunny yellow smoothie certainly is! Makes a great breakfast or snack and the tofu provides enough protein to help get you through to your next meal.

Unsweetened orange juice	2 cups	500 mL
Package of coconut dessert tofu	10 1/2 oz.	300 g
Frozen pineapple pieces	1 cup	250 mL
Frozen mango pieces	3/4 cup	175 mL

Process all 4 ingredients in blender until smooth. Makes about 4 cups (1 L). Serves 4.

1 serving: 179 Calories; 1.5 g Total Fat (0.1 g Mono, 0.1 g Poly, 0.2 g Sat); 0 mg Cholesterol; 40 g Carbohydrate; 2 g Fibre; 4 g Protein; 8 mg Sodium

CHOICES: 2 Fruits; 1/2 Meat & Alternatives

Pictured on page 54.

Veggie Pinwheels

These crisp and attractive tortilla spirals are filled with a warm filling of cream cheese and veggies. These taste just as good as they look!

Whole-wheat tortillas (9 inch, 22 cm, diameter)	2	2
Light garlic and herb cream cheese	1/3 cup	75 mL
Finely chopped celery	1/4 cup	60 mL
Finely chopped red pepper	1/4 cup	60 mL
Grated carrot	1/4 cup	60 mL
Pepper	1/4 tsp.	1 mL

Cooking spray

Preheat oven to 400°F (205°C). Place tortillas on work surface. Spread with cream cheese.

Sprinkle with next 4 ingredients. Roll up, jelly-roll style. Place, seam-side down, on ungreased baking sheet.

(continued on next page)

Spray with cooking spray. Bake for about 15 minutes until browned and crisp. Cut into 1 inch (2.5 cm) pieces. Makes about 14 pinwheels.

1 pinwheel: 26 Calories; 1.0 g Total Fat (0 g Mono, 0.2 g Poly, 0.6 g Sat); 4 mg Cholesterol; 4 g Carbohydrate; trace Fibre; 1 g Protein; 66 mg Sodium

CHOICES: None

Pictured on page 53.

Caramel Mocha Smoothie

You could start your morning with one of those expensive and high-calorie coffee house drinks—or you could make this healthier version yourself. A cool, sweet smoothie filled with the decadent flavours of coffee, chocolate and caramel.

Non-fat vanilla yogurt	2 cups	500 mL
Light hot chocolate mix	1/3 cup	75 mL
Cold strong prepared coffee	1/4 cup	60 mL
Caramel ice cream topping	1 tbsp.	15 mL

Process first 3 ingredients in blender or food processor until smooth. Makes about 2 1/2 cups (625 mL). Divide between 2 glasses.

Drizzle with ice cream topping. Serves 2.

1 serving: 366 Calories; trace Total Fat (trace Mono, 0 g Poly, trace Sat); 5 mg Cholesterol; 66 g Carbohydrate; 4 g Fibre; 22 g Protein; 839 mg Sodium

CHOICES: 1 1/2 Other Choices; 2 1/2 Milk & Alternatives

Pictured on page 54.

Paré Pointer
Bloodhounds are in the money. They're always picking up scents.

Orange Beef Capellini

Asian flavour takes an orange twist in this stir-fried one-dish meal.
Dress this dish up for company by adding a garnish of chopped
parsley and fresh orange segments.

Water	8 cups	2 L
Salt	1 tsp.	5 mL
Capellini pasta	8 oz.	225 g
Sesame (or canola) oil	2 tsp.	10 mL
Beef stir-fry strips	1 lb.	454 g
Fresh mixed stir-fry vegetables, larger pieces cut smaller	6 cups	1.5 L
Garlic cloves, minced (or 1/2 tsp., 2 mL, powder)	2	2
Finely grated gingerroot (or 1/2 tsp., 2 mL, ground ginger)	2 tsp.	10 mL
Prepared beef broth	1/2 cup	125 mL
Hoisin sauce	3 tbsp.	50 mL
Soy sauce	3 tbsp.	50 mL
Frozen concentrated orange juice	1/4 cup	60 mL
Cornstarch	1 tsp.	5 mL
Sesame oil (for flavour)	1 tsp.	5 mL

Combine water and salt in large saucepan or Dutch oven. Bring to a boil. Add pasta. Boil, uncovered, for 4 to 6 minutes, stirring occasionally, until tender but firm. Drain. Return to same pot. Cover to keep warm.

Meanwhile, heat first amount of sesame oil in large frying pan on medium-high. Add beef. Stir-fry for 1 minute. Add next 3 ingredients. Stir-fry for about 5 minutes until vegetables start to soften.

Combine remaining 6 ingredients in small bowl. Add to beef mixture. Cook for about 2 minutes, stirring occasionally, until sauce is boiling and slightly thickened and vegetables are tender-crisp. Add pasta. Toss until coated. Makes about 8 cups (2 L). Serves 4.

1 serving: 580 Calories; 12.7 g Total Fat (4.0 g Mono, 1.8 g Poly, 3.4 g Sat); 43 mg Cholesterol; 76 g Carbohydrate; 3 g Fibre; 38 g Protein; 1815 mg Sodium

CHOICES: 3 Grains & Starches; 1/2 Fruits; 4 Vegetables; 3 Meat & Alternatives; 1/2 Fats

Pictured on page 71.

Apricot Beef Stir-Fry

*You'll have no beefs with this tasty stir-fry of beef,
broccoli and sweet dried apricots.*

Cornstarch	2 tsp.	10 mL
Prepared beef broth	1 tbsp.	15 mL
Prepared beef broth	1 cup	250 mL
Garlic powder	1/2 tsp.	2 mL
Ground cumin	1/2 tsp.	2 mL
Ground ginger	1/2 tsp.	2 mL
Ground cinnamon	1/4 tsp.	1 mL
Pepper	1/4 tsp.	1 mL
Canola oil	2 tsp.	10 mL
Beef top sirloin steak, trimmed of fat and thinly sliced	1 lb.	454 mL
Broccoli florets	2 cups	500 mL
Chopped dried apricot	1/4 cup	60 mL
Grated orange zest	2 tsp.	10 mL

Stir cornstarch into first amount of broth in small cup. Set aside.

Combine next 6 ingredients in small bowl. Set aside.

Heat large frying pan or wok on medium-high until very hot. Add canola oil. Add beef. Stir-fry for about 2 minutes until no longer pink. Remove to small bowl with slotted spoon. Cover to keep warm. Reduce heat to medium.

Add broccoli and apricot to same frying pan. Stir-fry for 1 minute. Add broth mixture. Cook, covered, for about 3 minutes, stirring occasionally, until broccoli is tender-crisp. Stir cornstarch mixture. Add to broccoli mixture. Heat and stir for 1 to 2 minutes until boiling and thickened.

Add orange zest and beef. Stir. Makes about 4 cups (1 L). Serves 4.

1 serving: 238 Calories; 10.5 g Total Fat (4.7 g Mono, 1.0 g Poly, 3.3 g Sat); 60 mg Cholesterol; 10 g Carbohydrate; 2 g Fibre; 26 g Protein; 374 mg Sodium

CHOICES: 1/2 Fruits; 3 1/2 Meat & Alternatives; 1/2 Fats

Dijon Beef On Rye

Dijon mustard and caraway seed flavour a warm, creamy beef stew served on toasted rye bread. Try it on caraway rye bread for even more flavour. Serve with a crisp salad for a complete meal.

Canola oil	1 tsp.	5 mL
Beef stir-fry strips, cut into 1 inch (2.5 cm) pieces	1 lb.	454 g
Chopped fresh white mushrooms	1 1/2 cups	375 mL
Chopped onion	1/2 cup	125 mL
Diced celery	1/2 cup	125 mL
Garlic clove, minced (or 1/4 tsp., 1 mL, powder)	1	1
All-purpose flour	3 tbsp.	50 mL
Can of skim evaporated milk	13 1/2 oz.	385 mL
Frozen cut green beans, thawed	1 1/2 cups	375 mL
Dijon mustard	1 1/2 tbsp.	25 mL
Caraway seed	3/4 tsp.	4 mL
Salt	1/2 tsp.	2 mL
Pepper	1/4 tsp.	1 mL
Rye bread slices	4	4
Dijon mustard	4 tsp.	20 mL

Heat canola oil in large frying pan on medium-high. Add next 5 ingredients. Scramble-fry for about 7 minutes until celery is softened.

Sprinkle flour over beef mixture. Heat and stir for 1 minute.

Add milk. Heat and stir until boiling and thickened. Add next 5 ingredients. Cook and stir until heated through.

Toast bread slices. Spread with mustard. Transfer to 4 plates. Spoon beef mixture over toast slices. Serves 4.

1 serving: 390 Calories; 10.0 g Total Fat (4.5 g Mono, 1.0 g Poly, 3.0 g Sat); 73 mg Cholesterol; 37 g Carbohydrate; 4 g Fibre; 36 g Protein; 838 mg Sodium

CHOICES: 1 Grains & Starches; 1 Vegetables; 1/2 Milk & Alternatives; 3 Meat & Alternatives

Pictured on page 72.

Beef & Pork

Greek Beef Burritos

Opa meets olé! Try burritos with a Greek twist for dinner tonight. For even quicker prep, set bowls of the beef and toppings on the table and have everybody assemble their own burritos.

Flour tortillas (9 inch, 22 cm, diameter)	4	4
Beef top sirloin steak	1 lb.	454 g
Greek seasoning, sprinkle		
Low-fat plain yogurt	1/4 cup	60 mL
Chopped fresh basil	2 tbsp.	30 mL
Sliced red onion	1/4 cup	60 mL
Shredded lettuce, lightly packed	1 cup	250 mL
Chopped tomato	1/2 cup	125 mL
Crumbled feta cheese	1/2 cup	125 mL
Can of sliced black olives, drained	4 1/2 oz.	128 mL

Wrap tortillas in foil. Preheat gas barbecue to medium-high (see Tip, page 77). Place tortillas on ungreased grill. Turn burner under tortillas to low and leave opposite burner on medium-high. Close lid. Cook for about 10 minutes until warmed.

Meanwhile, sprinkle both sides of steak with Greek seasoning. Cook steak on greased grill for about 5 minutes per side until desired doneness. Remove to plate. Cover with foil. Let stand for 5 minutes.

Combine yogurt and basil in small cup.

Layer remaining 5 ingredients, in order given, on warmed tortillas. Thinly slice steak. Arrange over olives. Drizzle with yogurt mixture. Fold bottom ends of tortillas over filling. Fold in sides. Fold over from bottom to enclose filling. Makes 4 burritos.

1 burrito: 398 Calories; 17.9 g Total Fat (5.8 g Mono, 0.6 g Poly, 6.2 g Sat); 69 mg Cholesterol; 27 g Carbohydrate; 2 g Fibre; 31 g Protein; 787 mg Sodium

CHOICES: 1 1/2 Grains & Starches; 3 Meat & Alternatives; 1/2 Fats

Peppered Beef

This lively stir-fry is peppered with, well—peppers! Sliced bell peppers, seasoned with black and cayenne pepper. A terrific topper for rice, noodles or even mashed potatoes.

Low-sodium beef broth	1/2 cup	125 mL
Low-sodium soy sauce	1/4 cup	60 mL
Cornstarch	1 tbsp.	15 mL
Garlic powder	1/2 tsp.	2 mL
Pepper	1/2 tsp.	2 mL
Cayenne pepper	1/8 tsp.	0.5 mL
Canola oil	1 tsp.	5 mL
Thinly sliced green pepper	1 1/2 cups	375 mL
Thinly sliced red pepper	1 1/2 cups	375 mL
Sliced fresh white mushrooms	2 cups	500 mL
Canola oil	2 tsp.	10 mL
Beef stir-fry strips	3/4 lb.	340 g

Combine first 6 ingredients in small bowl. Set aside.

Heat wok or large frying pan on medium-high until very hot. Add first amount of canola oil. Add green and red peppers. Stir-fry for 1 minute. Add mushrooms. Stir-fry for about 2 minutes until peppers are tender-crisp. Remove vegetables to plate. Cover to keep warm.

Heat second amount of canola oil in same wok. Add beef. Stir-fry for about 2 minutes until starting to brown. Add broth mixture. Heat and stir for about 1 minute until sauce is boiling and thickened. Add vegetables. Stir. Makes about 4 cups (1 L). Serves 4.

1 serving: 206 Calories; 8.6 g Total Fat (4.2 g Mono, 1.4 g Poly, 2.1 g Sat); 52 mg Cholesterol; 11 g Carbohydrate; 2 g Fibre; 21 g Protein; 551 mg Sodium

CHOICES: 1 Vegetables; 2 1/2 Meat & Alternatives; 1/2 Fats

Apricot Ginger Pork

Rich, sweet apricot and ginger does double-duty as an attractive glaze and a dipping sauce for flavourful pork.

Pork tenderloin, trimmed of fat	1 lb.	454 g
Cooking spray		
Seasoned salt	1/2 tsp.	2 mL
Apricot jam	1/2 cup	125 mL
Apple cider vinegar	2 tbsp.	30 mL
Liquid honey	1 tbsp.	15 mL
Low-sodium soy sauce	1 tbsp.	15 mL
Finely grated gingerroot (or 1/2 tsp., 2 mL, ground ginger)	2 tsp.	10 mL
Garlic powder	1/4 tsp.	1 mL

Preheat oven to 475°F (240°C). Place tenderloin on greased wire rack set on foil-lined baking sheet. Spray with cooking spray. Sprinkle with seasoned salt. Bake for 20 minutes.

Meanwhile, combine remaining 6 ingredients in small saucepan. Bring to a boil. Simmer, uncovered, for about 7 minutes, stirring occasionally, until thickened. Measure 3 tbsp. (50 mL) jam mixture into small cup. Brush over pork. Reserve remaining jam mixture. Bake pork for about 5 minutes until meat thermometer inserted into thickest part of tenderloin reads 155°F (68°C). Transfer to serving dish. Cover with foil. Let stand for 10 minutes. Internal temperature should rise to at least 160°F (70°C). Serve with reserved jam mixture. Serves 4.

1 serving: 264 Calories; 4.9 g Total Fat (2.2 g Mono, 0.5 g Poly, 1.7 g Sat); 71 mg Cholesterol; 31 g Carbohydrate; trace Fibre; 24 g Protein; 370 mg Sodium

CHOICES: 2 Other Choices; 3 Meat & Alternatives

Paré Pointer
If you have a copper ore, you need a copper boat to go with it.

Raspberry Steak

Tangy-sweet raspberries and perfectly cooked steak make this a truly decadent, yet surprisingly light dinner option.

Olive (or canola) oil	1 tbsp.	15 mL
Beef top sirloin steak	1 lb.	454 g
Salt	1/4 tsp.	1 mL
Pepper	1/2 tsp.	2 mL
Fresh (or frozen whole) raspberries	3/4 cup	175 mL
Water	1/4 cup	60 mL
Liquid honey	2 tbsp.	30 mL
Tub margarine	1 tbsp.	15 mL
Ground cinnamon	1/2 tsp.	2 mL
Ground ginger	1/4 tsp.	1 mL
Balsamic vinegar	2 tsp.	10 mL

Heat olive oil in large frying pan on medium-high. Sprinkle both sides of steak with salt and pepper. Add to frying pan. Cook for 3 to 4 minutes per side until desired doneness. Transfer to cutting board. Cover with foil. Let stand for 5 minutes.

Meanwhile, reduce heat to medium. Add next 6 ingredients to same frying pan. Heat and stir until boiling. Simmer for about 4 minutes until sauce starts to thicken.

Add vinegar. Stir. Slice steak diagonally across the grain into 1/4 inch (6 mm) thick slices. Serve sauce over beef. Serves 4.

1 serving: 267 Calories; 13.9 g Total Fat (6.9 g Mono, 2.4 g Poly, 3.6 g Sat); 67 mg Cholesterol; 12 g Carbohydrate; 2 g Fibre; 22 g Protein; 238 mg Sodium

CHOICES: 1/2 Other Choices; 3 Meat & Alternatives

Pictured on front cover.

Portuguese Pork Chops

A versatile Portuguese-inspired sauce of tomatoes, olives and clams served with tender pork chops. The sauce is also great over rice, pasta or green beans.

Olive (or canola) oil	2 tsp.	10 mL
Boneless pork loin chops, trimmed of fat (about 4 oz., 113 g, each)	6	6
Olive (or canola) oil	2 tsp.	10 mL
Chopped onion	1 cup	250 mL
Garlic clove, minced (or 1/4 tsp., 1 mL, powder)	1	1
Chopped red pepper	1 cup	250 mL
Can of diced tomatoes (with juice)	14 oz.	398 mL
Can of sliced black olives, drained	4 1/2 oz.	125 mL
Reserved clam liquid	1/2 cup	125 mL
Red wine vinegar	1/4 cup	60 mL
Tomato paste (see Tip, page 120)	3 tbsp.	50 mL
Paprika	1 tsp.	5 mL
Cayenne pepper	1/4 tsp.	1 mL
Pepper	1/8 tsp.	0.5 mL
Can of whole baby clams, drained and liquid reserved	5 oz.	142 g
Chopped fresh parsley	1/2 cup	125 mL

Heat first amount of olive oil in large frying pan on medium. Add pork chops. Cook for 2 to 3 minutes per side until browned. Remove to plate. Cover to keep warm.

Heat second amount of olive oil in same frying pan on medium. Add next 3 ingredients. Cook for about 5 minutes, stirring often, until softened.

Add next 8 ingredients. Stir. Bring to a boil.

Add clams and pork chops. Reduce heat to low. Cook, covered, for about 5 minutes until pork is no longer pink inside.

Add parsley. Stir. Serves 6.

1 serving: 298 Calories; 14.4 g Total Fat (7.4 g Mono, 1.6 g Poly, 3.8 g Sat); 91 mg Cholesterol; 12 g Carbohydrate; 2 g Fibre; 31 g Protein; 571 mg Sodium

CHOICES: 1 Vegetables; 4 Meat & Alternatives; 1/2 Fats

Grilled Caesar Burgers

This burger's got all the flavours of the classic salad. Try serving in your favourite crusty rolls, or add soy-based imitation bacon bits for smoky flavour without adding fat.

Garlic and herb croutons	1 cup	250 mL
Light Caesar dressing	1/2 cup	125 mL
Quick-cooking rolled oats	1/3 cup	75 mL
Lean ground beef	1 lb.	454 g
Shredded romaine lettuce, lightly packed	4 cups	1 L
Light Caesar dressing	1/4 cup	60 mL
Whole-wheat bread slices	4	4

Preheat gas barbecue to medium. Process croutons in blender or food processor until coarse crumbs form. Transfer to large bowl. Add first amount of dressing and oats. Stir. Add beef. Mix well. Divide into 4 equal portions. Shape into four 4 inch (10 cm) diameter patties. Cook on greased grill for about 7 minutes per side until fully cooked and internal temperature reaches 160°F (70°C).

Combine lettuce and second amount of dressing in medium bowl. Spoon onto bread slices. Top with patties. Makes 4 burgers.

1 burger: 438 Calories; 21.2 g Total Fat (8.9 g Mono, 2.1 g Poly, 7.3 g Sat); 69 mg Cholesterol; 34 g Carbohydrate; 4 g Fibre; 28 g Protein; 835 mg Sodium

CHOICES: 1 1/2 Grains & Starches; 3 Meat & Alternatives

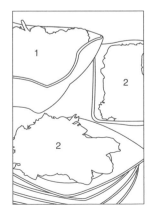

1. Orange Beef Capellini, page 62
2. Herb-Rubbed Pork Tenderloin, page 77

Props courtesy of: Danesco Inc.

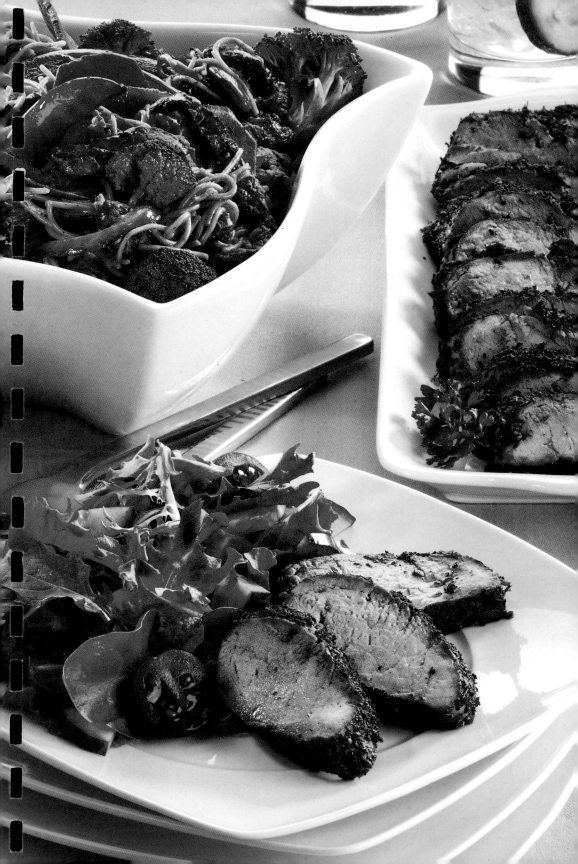

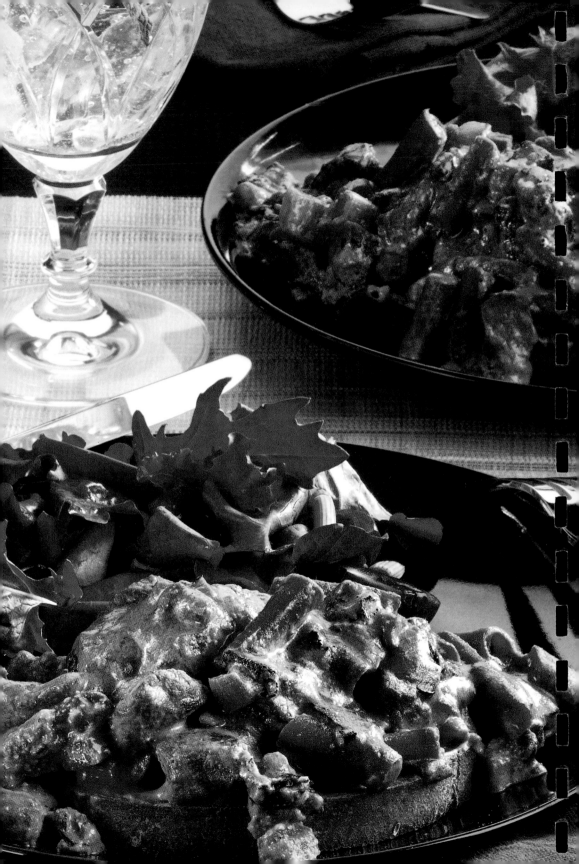

Curried Fruit Pork Chops

Enjoy the exotic spices of curry—without the rich and heavy sauces that usually go along with it. A fresh medley of tropical fruit adds lots of flavour to these juicy chops.

Curry powder	1 tbsp.	15 mL
Salt	1/2 tsp.	2 mL
Boneless centre-cut pork chops, trimmed of fat	4	4
Canola oil	2 tsp.	10 mL
Diced banana	1 cup	250 mL
Diced fresh pineapple	1 cup	250 mL
Diced ripe mango	1 cup	250 mL
Unsweetened applesauce	1/4 cup	60 mL

Combine curry powder and salt in small cup. Sprinkle over both sides of pork chops.

Heat canola oil in large frying pan on medium-high. Add pork chops. Cook for 1 to 2 minutes per side until browned. Reduce heat to medium-low.

Add remaining 4 ingredients. Stir. Cook, covered, for about 4 minutes, stirring at halftime, until pork is no longer pink inside. Serves 4.

1 serving: 346 Calories; 16.9 g Total Fat (7.5 g Mono, 2.4 g Poly, 5.4 g Sat); 78 mg Cholesterol; 23 g Carbohydrate; 3 g Fibre; 26 g Protein; 363 mg Sodium

CHOICES: 1 1/2 Fruits; 3 1/2 Meat & Alternatives; 1/2 Fats

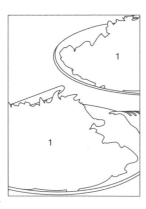

1. Dijon Beef On Rye, page 64

Pork Apple Skillet

An Oktoberfest special! The traditional German flavours of sauerkraut and caraway, sweetened with apple. A perfect accompaniment to tender, golden-brown pork chops.

Canola oil	2 tsp.	10 mL
Boneless fast-fry pork chops (about 4 oz., 113 g, each)	6	6
Pepper	1/2 tsp.	2 mL
Sliced fresh white mushrooms	2 cups	500 mL
Sliced onion	1 1/2 cups	375 mL
Medium peeled cooking apples (such as McIntosh), sliced	2	2
Caraway seed	1 tsp.	5 mL
Jar of wine sauerkraut, drained	17 1/2 oz.	500 mL
Can of diced tomatoes (with juice)	14 oz.	398 mL

Heat canola oil in large frying pan on medium-high. Add pork chops to frying pan. Sprinkle with pepper. Cook for about 2 minutes per side until browned and no longer pink. Remove to plate. Cover to keep warm.

Add mushrooms to same frying pan. Cook and stir for about 1 minute until mushrooms start to release liquid. Add next 3 ingredients. Reduce heat to medium. Cook for about 3 minutes, stirring occasionally, until onion starts to soften.

Add sauerkraut and tomatoes. Cook and stir for about 2 minutes until heated through. Serve with pork chops. Serves 6.

1 serving: 247 Calories; 8.2 g Total Fat (3.8 g Mono, 1.0 g Poly, 2.5 g Sat); 65 mg Cholesterol; 18 g Carbohydrate; 4 g Fibre; 26 g Protein; 778 mg Sodium

CHOICES: 1/2 Fruits; 1 Vegetables; 3 Meat & Alternatives

Ginger Wasabi Skewers

Japanese flavours of pickled ginger, mirin and wasabi transform meatball skewers into something extraordinary. Use the leftover green onion tops for salads, soups or pasta.

WASABI MAYONNAISE

Mayonnaise (not salad dressing)	1/2 cup	125 mL
Wasabi paste (Japanese horseradish)	2 tsp.	10 mL

MEATBALL SKEWERS

Large egg, fork-beaten	1	1
Crushed soda crackers	1/2 cup	125 mL
Finely chopped pickled ginger slices	2 tbsp.	30 mL
Soy sauce	2 tbsp.	30 mL
Thinly sliced green onion (green part only)	2 tbsp.	30 mL
Mirin (Japanese sweet cooking seasoning)	1 tbsp.	15 mL
Lean ground beef	1 lb.	454 g
Pickled ginger slices, larger slices folded in half	24	24
Green onions (white part only), cut into 2 inch (5 cm) pieces	24	24
Bamboo skewers (8 inches, 20 cm, each), soaked in water for 10 minutes	8	8

Wasabi Mayonnaise: Combine mayonnaise and wasabi paste in small bowl. Chill. Makes about 1/2 cup (125 mL) mayonnaise.

Meatball Skewers: Preheat gas barbecue to medium (see Tip, page 77). Combine first 6 ingredients in large bowl. Add beef. Mix well. Roll into 32 balls, about 1 inch (2.5 cm) diameter each.

Thread meatballs and second amounts of ginger slices and green onion alternately onto skewers, beginning and ending with meatballs. Cook skewers on greased grill for about 14 minutes, turning occasionally, until meatballs are no longer pink inside and internal temperature reaches 160°F (71°C). Serve with Wasabi Mayonnaise. Makes 8 skewers. Serves 4.

1 serving: 556 Calories; 39.9 g Total Fat (8.1 g Mono, 0.8 g Poly, 9.8 g Sat); 124 mg Cholesterol; 19 g Carbohydrate; 3 g Fibre; 27 g Protein; 879 mg Sodium

CHOICES: 1/2 Grains & Starches; 1 Vegetables; 3 Meat & Alternatives; 4 Fats

Lemon Grass Beef

If you're looking for a ground beef recipe that's just a little different, try this lovely, light curry that goes great over rice or pasta.

Canola oil	1 tsp.	5 mL
Extra-lean ground beef	1 lb.	454 g
Chopped onion	1 cup	250 mL
Frozen sliced carrot	2 cups	500 mL
Chopped red pepper	1 cup	250 mL
Lime juice	2 tbsp.	30 mL
Soy sauce	2 tbsp.	30 mL
Brown sugar, packed	1 tbsp.	15 mL
Finely chopped lemon grass, bulb only (root and stalk removed)	1 tbsp.	15 mL
Garlic cloves, minced (or 1/2 tsp., 2 mL, powder)	2	2
Finely grated gingerroot	1 tsp.	5 mL
Red curry paste	1/4 tsp.	1 mL
All-purpose flour	1 tbsp.	15 mL
Light coconut milk	1/2 cup	125 mL
Chopped fresh cilantro	2 tsp.	10 mL

Heat canola oil in large frying pan on medium-high. Add beef and onion. Scramble-fry for 5 to 10 minutes until beef is no longer pink. Drain.

Add next 9 ingredients. Cook for about 5 minutes, stirring occasionally, until red pepper is tender-crisp.

Sprinkle with flour. Heat and stir for 1 minute.

Add coconut milk. Heat and stir for about 1 minute until boiling and thickened.

Sprinkle with cilantro. Makes about 5 cups (1.25 L). Serves 4.

1 serving: 281 Calories; 10.8 g Total Fat (3.8 g Mono, 0.6 g Poly, 4.9 g Sat); 60 mg Cholesterol; 19 g Carbohydrate; 3 g Fibre; 26 g Protein; 521 mg Sodium

CHOICES: 2 Vegetables; 3 Meat & Alternatives

Herb-Rubbed Pork Tenderloin

Grilled pork tenderloin is both lean and delicious, but the secret to cooking up juicy, tender pork on the barbecue is being careful not to overcook it! The flavourful herbs and spices make this recipe truly unforgettable.

Pork tenderloin, trimmed of fat	1 lb.	454 g
Canola oil	1 tbsp.	15 mL
Dried basil	1 tbsp.	15 mL
Dried oregano	1 tbsp.	15 mL
Dried parsley flakes	1 tbsp.	15 mL
Chili powder	2 tsp.	10 mL
Garlic powder	1 tsp.	5 mL
Salt	1/2 tsp.	2 mL
Coarsely ground pepper	1 tsp.	5 mL

Preheat gas barbecue to medium (see Tip, below). Brush tenderloin with canola oil.

Combine next 7 ingredients in small bowl. Rub over surface of tenderloin. Cook on greased grill for about 20 minutes, turning occasionally, until meat thermometer inserted into thickest part of tenderloin reads 155°F (68°C). Remove from grill and transfer to cutting board. Cover with foil. Let stand for 10 minutes. Internal temperature should rise to at least 160°F (70°C). Cut into 1/2 inch (12 mm) slices. Serves 4.

1 serving: 190 Calories; 8.5 g Total Fat (4.2 g Mono, 1.6 g Poly, 1.9 g Sat); 71 mg Cholesterol; 3 g Carbohydrate; 1 g Fibre; 25 g Protein; 365 mg Sodium

CHOICES: 3 Meat & Alternatives; 1/2 Fats

Pictured on page 71.

 tip Too cold to barbecue? Use the broiler instead! Your food should cook in about the same length of time—and remember to turn or baste as directed. Set your oven rack so that the food is about 3 to 4 inches (7.5 to 10 cm) away from the top element—for most ovens, this is the top rack.

White Chicken Chili

*Chili without tomatoes? Why not? The absence of heavy tomato flavour lets
your taste buds focus on the subtle taste of chili, lime and cilantro.*

Canola oil	2 tsp.	10 mL
All-purpose flour	1/4 cup	60 mL
Chili powder	2 tsp.	10 mL
Garlic powder	1/2 tsp.	2 mL
Ground cumin	1/2 tsp.	2 mL
Boneless, skinless chicken thighs, cut into 1 inch (2.5 cm) pieces	1 lb.	454 g
Sliced fresh white mushrooms	2 cups	500 mL
Chopped onion	1/2 cup	125 mL
Low-sodium prepared chicken broth	1 1/2 cups	375 mL
Can of white kidney beans, rinsed and drained	19 oz.	540 mL
Chopped fresh cilantro	3 tbsp.	50 mL
Sliced green onion	2 tbsp.	30 mL
Lime juice	4 tsp.	20 mL

Heat canola oil in large saucepan on medium-high. Combine next
4 ingredients in large resealable freezer bag. Add chicken. Toss until
coated. Add chicken to pan, reserving any remaining flour mixture. Cook,
uncovered, for about 5 minutes, stirring occasionally, until browned on all
sides. Remove to plate. Cover to keep warm.

Add mushrooms and onion to same saucepan. Cook for about 3 minutes,
stirring often, until onion is softened. Add chicken and reserved flour
mixture. Heat and stir for 1 minute.

Slowly add broth, stirring constantly until smooth. Heat and stir until
boiling and thickened. Add beans. Stir. Reduce heat to medium-low. Cook,
covered, for about 3 minutes until heated through.

Add remaining 3 ingredients. Stir. Makes about 4 3/4 cups (1.2 L). Serves 4.

*1 serving: 342 Calories; 12.2 g Total Fat (4.6 g Mono, 2.7 g Poly, 2.6 g Sat); 76 mg Cholesterol;
28 g Carbohydrate; 6 g Fibre; 29 g Protein; 352 mg Sodium*

CHOICES: 1 Grains & Starches; 3 1/2 Meat & Alternatives

Pictured on page 89.

Country Herb Turkey

Basil and lemon pepper lend a refreshing tanginess to this medley of turkey and fresh vegetables. Serve over pasta, rice or mashed potatoes.

Canola oil	1 tbsp.	15 mL
Turkey scaloppine	8	8
(about 2 oz., 57 g, each)		
Lemon pepper, sprinkle		
Chopped onion	1 cup	250 mL
Chopped carrot	1/2 cup	125 mL
Chopped celery	1/2 cup	125 mL
Dried thyme	1/2 tsp.	2 mL
All-purpose flour	2 tbsp.	30 mL
Low-sodium prepared chicken broth	2 cups	500 mL
Basil pesto	1 tbsp.	15 mL

Heat 1 tsp. (5 mL) canola oil in large frying pan on medium-high. Sprinkle turkey with lemon pepper. Add to frying pan. Cook, in 4 batches, for about 30 seconds per side, until no longer pink inside, adding 1 tsp. (5 mL) canola oil for each batch. Remove to plate. Cover to keep warm. Reduce heat to medium.

Add next 4 ingredients to same frying pan. Cook, covered, for about 2 minutes until vegetables start to soften.

Sprinkle with flour. Heat and stir for 1 minute. Slowly add broth, stirring constantly until boiling and thickened.

Add pesto. Stir. Cook for about 5 minutes until vegetables are tender. Add turkey. Cook for about 1 minute until turkey is heated through. Serves 4.

1 serving: 216 Calories; 7.0 g Total Fat (2.0 g Mono, 1.1 g Poly, 0.6 g Sat); 48 mg Cholesterol; 10 g Carbohydrate; 1 g Fibre; 30 g Protein; 422 mg Sodium

CHOICES: 1 Vegetables; 4 Meat & Alternatives; 1 Fats

Pictured on page 89.

Coconut Chicken Curry

This spicy coconut curry is the perfect way to jazz up your weekday dinner with a little exotic flair. Spoon the sauce over basmati or jasmine rice.

Canola oil	1 tbsp.	15 mL
Boneless, skinless chicken thighs, cut into 1 inch (2.5 cm) cubes	1 lb.	454 g
Salt, sprinkle		
Pepper, sprinkle		
Can of chickpeas (garbanzo beans), rinsed and drained	19 oz.	540 mL
Can of light coconut milk	14 oz.	398 mL
Can of stewed tomatoes	14 oz.	398 mL
Dark raisins	1/4 cup	60 mL
Hot Madras curry paste	2 tbsp.	30 mL
Garlic cloves, minced (or 3/4 tsp., 4 mL, powder)	3	3
Finely grated gingerroot	1 tbsp.	15 mL
Brown sugar, packed	2 tsp.	10 mL
Chopped fresh cilantro	2 tbsp.	30 mL

Heat canola oil in large frying pan on medium-high. Add chicken. Sprinkle with salt and pepper. Cook for about 5 minutes, stirring occasionally, until starting to brown. Drain.

Add next 8 ingredients. Stir. Bring to a boil. Reduce heat to medium. Boil gently, uncovered, for about 12 minutes, stirring often, until chicken is no longer pink inside and sauce is slightly thickened.

Sprinkle with cilantro. Makes about 5 1/2 cups (1.4 L). Serves 6.

1 serving: 312 Calories; 14.7 g Total Fat (3.9 g Mono, 2.7 g Poly, 5.4 g Sat); 50 mg Cholesterol; 25 g Carbohydrate; 4 g Fibre; 19 g Protein; 484 mg Sodium

CHOICES: 1/2 Grains & Starches; 1/2 Fruits; 2 Meat & Alternatives

Chicken Lettuce Wraps

Cut the carbs by replacing tortillas with lettuce leaves in these sweet and spicy Asian-flavoured wraps. Use the large outside leaves from a head of green leaf lettuce, or overlap two smaller leaves.

Sesame (or canola) oil	2 tsp.	10 mL
Boneless, skinless chicken breast halves, cut into 1/4 inch (6 mm) strips	1 lb.	454 g
Garlic cloves, minced (or 1/2 tsp., 2 mL, powder)	2	2
Liquid honey	2 tbsp.	30 mL
Soy sauce	2 tbsp.	30 mL
Peanut butter	1 tbsp.	15 mL
Chili paste (sambal oelek)	1/2 tsp.	2 mL
Cooked long-grain brown rice (about 3/4 cups, 175 mL, uncooked)	2 cups	500 mL
Large green leaf lettuce leaves	8	8

Heat sesame oil in medium frying pan on medium. Add chicken and garlic. Cook for about 8 minutes, stirring occasionally, until chicken is no longer pink.

Add next 4 ingredients. Heat and stir for 2 minutes.

Add rice. Cook and stir for about 2 minutes until heated through. Makes about 3 1/2 cups (875 mL) filling.

Spoon about 6 tbsp. (100 mL) chicken mixture in centre of 1 leaf. Fold sides over filling. Roll up from bottom to enclose. Repeat with remaining chicken mixture and lettuce. Makes 8 wraps. Serves 4.

1 serving: 322 Calories; 7.0 g Total Fat (2.6 g Mono, 2.2 g Poly, 1.4 g Sat); 66 mg Cholesterol; 33 g Carbohydrate; 2 g Fibre; 30 g Protein; 482 mg Sodium

CHOICES: 1 1/2 Grains & Starches; 1/2 Other Choices; 3 Meat & Alternatives

Walnut Dijon-Crusted Chicken

Tender chicken dresses for success with a coating of crunchy walnuts, tangy Dijon and mildly sweet graham crumbs.

Dijon mustard	1/4 cup	60 mL
Boneless, skinless chicken breast halves (4 – 6 oz., 113 – 170 g, each)	4	4
Graham cracker crumbs	1/2 cup	125 mL
Ground walnuts	1/2 cup	125 mL
Tub margarine, melted	2 tbsp.	30 mL
Ground coriander	1/2 tsp.	2 mL
Ground ginger	1/2 tsp.	2 mL
Salt	1/4 tsp.	1 mL

Preheat oven to 425°F (220°C). Brush mustard on both sides of each chicken breast.

Combine remaining 6 ingredients in medium shallow dish. Press both sides of each chicken breast into crumb mixture until coated. Place on greased baking sheet. Bake for about 20 minutes until golden and internal temperature reaches 170°F (77°C). Serves 4.

1 serving: 167 Calories; 5.2 g Total Fat (1.4 g Mono, 2.3 g Poly, 0.9 g Sat); 66 mg Cholesterol; 2 g Carbohydrate; trace Fibre; 26 g Protein; 328 mg Sodium

CHOICES: 4 Meat & Alternatives

Baked Italian Patties

These hearty patties may be short on ingredients, but they're long on flavour! No burger buns are required, just a tossed green salad and a side of pasta.

Large egg, fork-beaten	1	1
Fine dry bread crumbs	1/3 cup	75 mL
Sun-dried tomato pesto	2 tbsp.	30 mL
Italian seasoning	1 tsp.	5 mL
Lean ground chicken breast	1 lb.	454 g
Tomato sauce	1/4 cup	60 mL
Grated Italian cheese blend	6 tbsp.	100 mL

(continued on next page)

Preheat oven to 400°F (205°C). Combine first 4 ingredients in medium bowl. Add chicken. Mix well. Divide into 4 equal portions. Shape into 1/2 inch (12 mm) thick oval patties. Arrange on greased baking sheet. Bake for about 12 minutes until fully cooked and internal temperature reaches 175°F (80°C).

Spread tomato sauce over patties. Sprinkle with cheese. Bake for about 3 minutes until cheese is melted. Makes 4 patties.

1 patty: 240 Calories; 6.2 g Total Fat (1.2 g Mono, 0.7 g Poly, 2.7 g Sat); 120 mg Cholesterol; 12 g Carbohydrate; 1 g Fibre; 32 g Protein; 626 mg Sodium

CHOICES: 1/2 Grains & Starches; 3 1/2 Meat & Alternatives

Pineapple Chicken

A quick and delicious chicken dish with great sweet-and-sour flavour. Best served over jasmine rice.

Sesame (or canola) oil	1 tsp.	5 mL
Boneless, skinless chicken breast halves, cut into 1/4 inch (6 mm) strips	1 lb.	454 g
Garlic clove, minced (or 1/4 tsp., 1 mL, powder)	1	1
Soy sauce	1 tbsp.	15 mL
Can of pineapple chunks, drained	14 oz.	398 mL
Unsweetened applesauce	1/2 cup	125 mL
Sweet-and-sour sauce	1/4 cup	60 mL
Chopped green onion	2 tbsp.	30 mL

Heat sesame oil in large frying pan on medium. Add chicken. Cook for 5 minutes, stirring occasionally.

Add garlic and soy sauce. Cook for about 5 minutes, stirring occasionally, until chicken is no longer pink.

Add next 3 ingredients. Heat and stir for about 2 minutes until boiling.

Add green onion. Stir. Makes about 3 cups (750 mL). Serves 4.

1 serving: 236 Calories; 3.1 g Total Fat (0.9 g Mono, 0.9 g Poly, 0.7 g Sat); 66 mg Cholesterol; 25 g Carbohydrate; 2 g Fibre; 27 g Protein; 267 mg Sodium

CHOICES: 1 Fruits; 3 1/2 Meat & Alternatives

Mushroom Turkey Scaloppine

Not all mushroom sauces are calorie-laden. These tender turkey slices are covered in a light and flavourful sauce with nary a drop of cream.

Package of dried porcini mushrooms	3/4 oz.	22 g
Boiling water	1 cup	250 mL
All-purpose flour	1/2 cup	125 mL
Salt	1/2 tsp.	2 mL
Pepper	1/2 tsp.	2 mL
Turkey scaloppine (about 2 oz., 57 g, each)	8	8
Olive (or canola) oil	4 tsp.	20 mL
Olive (or canola) oil	1 tsp.	5 mL
Finely chopped onion	1/2 cup	125 mL
Apple juice	1/4 cup	60 mL
White wine vinegar	2 tsp.	10 mL
Salt	1/4 tsp.	1 mL
Pepper	1/4 tsp.	1 mL
Chopped fresh parsley	1 tbsp.	15 mL

Put mushrooms into small heatproof bowl. Add boiling water. Stir. Let stand for about 5 minutes until softened. Drain, reserving 3/4 cup (175 mL) liquid. Chop mushrooms. Set aside.

Meanwhile, combine next 3 ingredients on a plate. Press both sides of turkey into flour mixture. Discard any remaining flour mixture.

Heat 1 tsp. (5 mL) of first amount of olive oil in large frying pan on medium-high. Cook turkey, in 4 batches, for about 30 seconds per side, until no longer pink inside, adding 1 tsp. (5 mL) olive oil for each batch. Transfer to plate. Cover to keep warm. Reduce heat to medium.

Heat second amount of olive oil in same frying pan. Add onion and mushrooms. Cook for about 3 minutes, stirring often, until onion is softened.

Add next 4 ingredients and reserved mushroom liquid. Bring to a boil. Simmer for about 2 minutes until thickened. Pour over turkey.

Sprinkle with parsley. Serves 4.

1 serving: 242 Calories; 7.4 g Total Fat (4.3 g Mono, 0.6 g Poly, 0.8 g Sat); 45 mg Cholesterol; 15 g Carbohydrate; 1 g Fibre; 31 g Protein; 434 mg Sodium

CHOICES: 1/2 Grains & Starches; 3 Meat & Alternatives; 1 Fats

Quick Kabobs

Somehow, food that's served on a stick just seems like more fun! With lots of colourful veggies, these are just as pretty as they are delicious.

Thick teriyaki basting sauce	1/4 cup	60 mL
Lemon juice	2 tbsp.	30 mL
Garlic cloves, minced	2	2
(or 1/2 tsp., 2 mL, powder)		
Pepper	1/2 tsp.	2 mL
Boneless, skinless chicken breast halves,	1 lb.	454 g
cut into 24 equal pieces		
Medium green pepper,	1	1
cut into 24 equal pieces		
Medium red pepper,	1	1
cut into 24 equal pieces		
Medium fresh whole white	16	16
mushrooms, stems removed		
Bamboo skewers (8 inches, 20 cm, each),	8	8
soaked in water for 10 minutes		

Preheat barbecue to medium (see Tip, page 77). Combine first 4 ingredients in small cup.

Thread next 4 ingredients alternately onto skewers. Brush with half of teriyaki mixture. Cook on greased grill for about 13 minutes, turning occasionally and brushing with remaining teriyaki mixture, until chicken is no longer pink inside. Makes 8 kabobs. Serves 4.

1 serving: 173 Calories; 2.1 g Total Fat (0.5 g Mono, 0.5 g Poly, 0.5 g Sat); 66 mg Cholesterol; 9 g Carbohydrate; 1 g Fibre; 29 g Protein; 759 mg Sodium

CHOICES: 3 1/2 Meat & Alternatives

Grilled Chicken Fajitas

First, grill the chicken, peppers and onions on the barbecue for a smoky flavour, then have everybody assemble their own fajita—now that's a time-saver! Be sure to lay the chicken thighs flat on the grill to speed up the cooking time.

Olive (or canola) oil	2 tbsp.	30 mL
Balsamic vinegar	1 tbsp.	15 mL
Dijon mustard	1 tsp.	5 mL
Garlic clove, minced	1	1
(or 1/4 tsp., 1 mL, powder)		
Ground cumin	1 tsp.	5 mL
Cayenne pepper	1/2 tsp.	2 mL
Boneless, skinless chicken thighs	1 lb.	454 g
Large red pepper, quartered	1	1
Large yellow pepper, quartered	1	1
Medium red onion, quartered	1	1
Whole-wheat flour tortillas	4	4
(9 inch, 22 cm, diameter)		
Light sour cream	1/2 cup	125 mL
Salsa	1/2 cup	125 mL
Chopped green onion	1/4 cup	60 mL

Preheat gas barbecue to medium-high. Combine first 6 ingredients in small bowl.

Arrange next 4 ingredients on greased grill. Brush with olive oil mixture. Cook for about 12 minutes, turning occasionally and brushing with remaining olive oil mixture, until peppers and onions are softened and internal temperature of chicken reaches 170°C (77°F). Transfer to plate. Cover with foil. Let stand for 5 minutes. Cut chicken, peppers and onions into strips. Transfer to bowl.

Arrange chicken and vegetables down center of each tortilla. Add remaining 3 ingredients. Fold up bottoms. Fold in sides, leaving top ends open. Serves 4.

1 serving: 405 Calories; 19.3 g Total Fat (8.2 g Mono, 3.7 g Poly, 4.8 g Sat); 84 mg Cholesterol; 32 g Carbohydrate; 4 g Fibre; 27 g Protein; 481 mg Sodium

CHOICES: 1 Grains & Starches; 1 Vegetables; 3 Meat & Alternatives; 1 Fats

Pictured on page 90.

Citrus Herb Turkey Kabobs

*Summery citrus and herb flavours make these kabobs a hit when it's
just too hot to turn on the stove.*

Orange juice	1/2 cup	125 mL
Lemon juice	3 tbsp.	50 mL
Lime juice	3 tbsp.	50 mL
Canola oil	1 tbsp.	15 mL
Liquid honey	1 tbsp.	15 mL
Italian seasoning	1 tsp.	5 mL
Chopped fresh cilantro	1 tbsp.	15 mL
Grated orange zest	1/2 tsp.	2 mL
Boneless, skinless turkey breast halves, cut into 1 inch (2.5 cm) cubes	1 lb.	454 g
Bamboo skewers (8 inches, 20 cm, each), soaked in water for 10 minutes	4	4
Salt, sprinkle		
Pepper, sprinkle		

Preheat gas barbecue to medium (see Tip, page 77). Combine first
6 ingredients in small saucepan. Bring to a boil. Boil gently, uncovered,
on medium for about 12 minutes, stirring often, until reduced by half.

Add cilantro and orange zest. Stir.

Meanwhile, thread turkey onto skewers. Sprinkle with salt and pepper.
Cook on greased grill for about 12 minutes, turning and brushing
occasionally with orange juice mixture, until turkey is fully cooked and no
longer pink inside. Makes 4 kabobs.

*1 kabob: 226 Calories; 8.0 g Total Fat (4.3 g Mono, 2.3 g Poly, 0.8 g Sat); 70 mg Cholesterol;
9 g Carbohydrate; 0.1 g Fibre; 28 g Protein; 56 mg Sodium*

CHOICES: 4 Meat & Alternatives; 1 Fats

Lemon Sage Turkey Patties

Want some sage advice? Add oatmeal to lean turkey burgers to eliminate dryness and sneak in some fibre, too! Sage and lemon add a fresh summery flavour.

Large flake rolled oats	1 cup	250 mL
Milk	1/3 cup	75 mL
Chopped fresh sage	1 tbsp.	15 mL
(or 3/4 tsp., 4 mL, dried)		
Grated lemon zest	1 tsp.	5 mL
Salt	1/2 tsp.	2 mL
Pepper	1/4 tsp.	1 mL
Extra-lean ground turkey breast	1 lb.	454 g

Combine oats and milk in large bowl. Let stand for 3 minutes.

Add next 4 ingredients. Stir. Add turkey. Mix well. Heat large frying pan on medium. Divide mixture into 4 equal portions. Shape into 4 1/2 inch (11 cm) diameter patties. Spray pan with cooking spray. Add patties. Cook for about 5 minutes per side until browned and internal temperature reaches 175°F (80°C). Makes 4 patties.

1 patty: 210 Calories; 3.0 g Total Fat (0.1 g Mono, 0 g Poly, 0.1 g Sat); 46 mg Cholesterol; 15 g Carbohydrate; 2 g Fibre; 32 g Protein; 368 mg Sodium

CHOICES: 1 Grains & Starches; 4 Meat & Alternatives

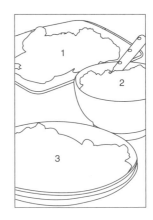

1. Rosemary Chicken Polenta, page 92
2. White Chicken Chili, page 78
3. Country Herb Turkey, page 79

Props courtesy of: Danesco Inc.
Wiltshire®

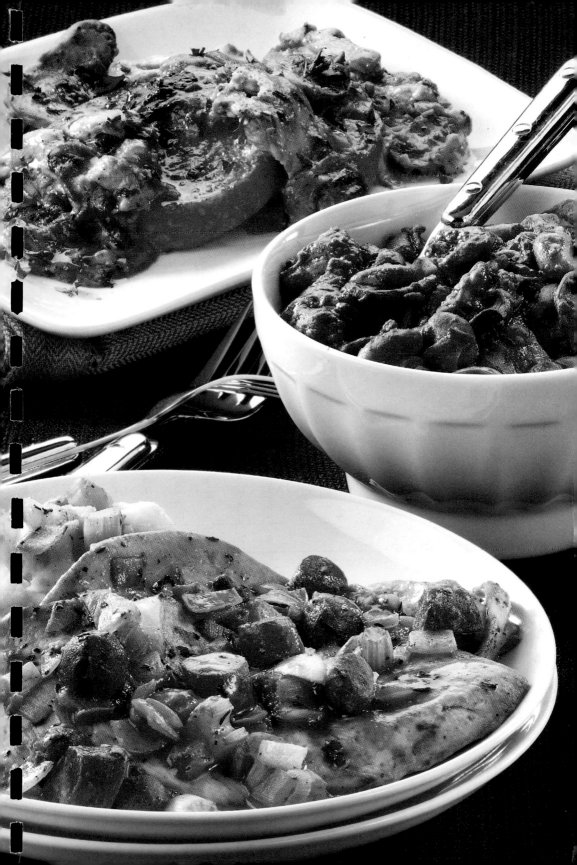

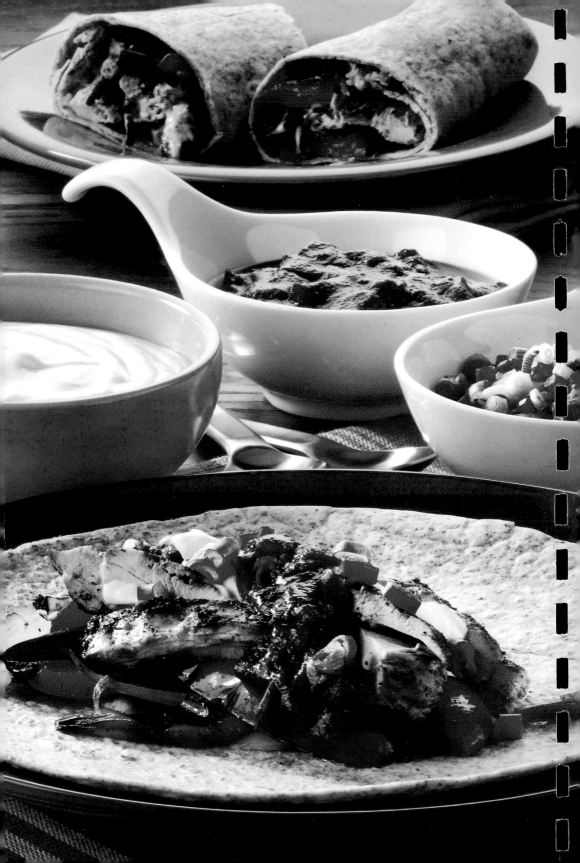

Mustard Dill Chicken

Tangy mustard chicken in a dill-y of a sauce! Serve with potatoes or egg noodles.

Canola oil	1 tbsp.	15 mL
Boneless, skinless chicken thighs	8	8
(about 3 oz., 85 g, each)		
Low-sodium prepared chicken broth	3/4 cup	175 mL
Dijon mustard (with whole seeds)	1 tbsp.	15 mL
Dried dillweed	1 tsp.	5 mL
Pepper	1/8 tsp.	0.5 mL
Milk	2 tbsp.	30 mL
Cornstarch	1 1/2 tsp.	7 mL

Heat canola oil in large frying pan on medium-high. Add chicken. Cook for 2 to 3 minutes per side until browned. Drain.

Add next 4 ingredients. Bring to a boil, stirring constantly and scraping any brown bits from bottom of pan. Reduce heat to medium. Boil gently, covered, for about 5 minutes until chicken is no longer pink inside.

Stir milk into cornstarch in small cup. Add to chicken mixture. Heat and stir for about 1 minute until boiling and thickened. Serves 4.

1 serving: 291 Calories; 16.6 g Total Fat (6.9 g Mono, 3.9 g Poly, 3.9 g Sat); 113 mg Cholesterol; 2 g Carbohydrate; trace Fibre; 31 g Protein; 297 mg Sodium

CHOICES: 4 Meat & Alternatives; 1/2 Fats

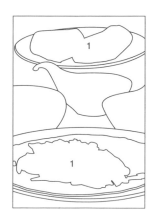

1. Grilled Chicken Fajitas, page 86

Props courtesy of: Danesco Inc.

Rosemary Chicken Polenta

*This creamy chicken and mushroom medley is served over dense, firm polenta
for a divinely different dinner.*

Canola oil	2 tsp.	10 mL
Boneless, skinless chicken breast halves, thinly sliced	1 lb.	454 g
Canola oil	2 tsp.	10 mL
Sliced fresh white mushrooms	2 cups	500 mL
Chopped onion	1 cup	250 mL
Chopped fresh rosemary (or 1/4 tsp., 1 mL, dried, crushed)	2 tsp.	10 mL
Garlic clove, minced (or 1/4 tsp., 1 mL, powder)	1	1
Salt	1/2 tsp.	2 mL
Pepper	1/4 tsp.	1 mL
All-purpose flour	3 tbsp.	50 mL
Can of 2% evaporated milk	13 1/2 oz.	385 mL
Grated lemon zest	1 tsp.	5 mL
Slices of prepared polenta roll, about 1/2 inch (12 mm) thick	8	8
Chopped fresh parsley	1 tbsp.	15 mL

Preheat broiler. Heat canola oil in large frying pan on medium-high. Add
chicken. Cook for about 5 minutes, stirring often, until no longer pink.
Remove to bowl. Cover to keep warm. Reduce heat to medium.

Heat second amount of canola oil in same frying pan. Add next 6 ingredients.
Cook for about 5 minutes, stirring often, until mushrooms and onion
are softened.

Add flour. Heat and stir for 1 minute. Slowly add evaporated milk, stirring
constantly until boiling and thickened. Add lemon zest and chicken. Stir.

Meanwhile, place polenta slices on greased baking sheet. Broil on top rack
in oven for about 3 minutes until golden. Remove to plate. Spoon chicken
mixture over polenta.

Sprinkle with parsley. Serves 4.

(continued on next page)

1 serving: 380 Calories; 8.4 g Total Fat (3.7 g Mono, 1.9 g Poly, 2.0 g Sat); 73 mg Cholesterol; 37 g Carbohydrate; 2 g Fibre; 37 g Protein; 817 mg Sodium

CHOICES: 1 1/2 Grains & Starches; 1 Vegetables; 1/2 Milk & Alternatives; 3 1/2 Meat & Alternatives; 1 Fats

Pictured on page 89.

Coconut Chicken

With the help of a few ingredients from your pantry, you'll have a delightful dinner with the smooth, light flavours of coconut and curry draped over tender chicken.

Boneless, skinless chicken breasts	6	6
(4 – 6 oz., 113 – 170 g, each)		
Cooking spray		
Can of light coconut milk	14 oz.	398 mL
All-purpose flour	2 tbsp.	30 mL
Brown sugar, packed	1 tbsp.	15 mL
Lime juice	1 tbsp.	15 mL
Soy sauce	1 tbsp.	15 mL
Thai red curry paste	1/2 tsp.	2 mL
Pepper	1/4 tsp.	1 mL

Preheat broiler. Arrange chicken in greased 9 x 9 inch (22 x 22 cm) baking dish. Spray with cooking spray. Broil on centre rack in oven for 5 minutes. Reduce heat to 450°F (230°C).

Meanwhile, whisk remaining 7 ingredients in small microwave-safe bowl until smooth. Microwave, covered, on high (100%) for about 2 minutes until hot. Carefully pour over chicken. Bake, uncovered, for about 12 minutes until chicken is fully cooked and internal temperature reaches 170°F (77°C). Serves 6.

1 serving: 196 Calories; 6.3 g Total Fat (0.5 g Mono, 0.4 g Poly, 3.8 g Sat); 66 mg Cholesterol; 6 g Carbohydrate; trace Fibre; 26 g Protein; 223 mg Sodium

CHOICES: 4 Meat & Alternatives

Basa With Mango Nut Salsa

Basa is a firm, mild fish that's definitely been gaining popularity. Its mild taste goes great with all sorts of flavours—like the freshness of mango, orange and lime.

MANGO NUT SALSA

Finely chopped frozen mango pieces, thawed	1 cup	250 mL
Finely chopped red pepper	1/4 cup	60 mL
Chopped whole hazelnuts (filberts), toasted (see Tip, page 114)	1/4 cup	60 mL
Chili powder	1 tbsp.	15 mL
Lime juice	1 tbsp.	15 mL
Frozen concentrated orange juice, thawed	2 tsp.	10 mL

LEMON PEPPER BASA

Canola oil	2 tsp.	10 mL
Basa fillets, cut into 4 equal portions	1 lb.	454 g
Lemon pepper	1/2 tsp.	2 mL
All-purpose flour	1/3 cup	75 mL

Mango Nut Salsa: Combine all 6 ingredients in small bowl. Makes about 1 cup (250 mL) salsa.

Lemon Pepper Basa: Heat canola oil in large frying pan on medium. Sprinkle both sides of fillets with lemon pepper. Press both sides of fillets into flour until coated. Discard any remaining flour. Add to frying pan. Cook for about 3 minutes per side until golden and fish flakes easily when tested with fork. Serve with Mango Nut Salsa. Serves 4.

1 serving: 242 Calories; 11.7 g Total Fat (4.7 g Mono, 1.4 g Poly, 2.3 g Sat); 51 mg Cholesterol; 19 g Carbohydrate; 2 g Fibre; 17 g Protein; 118 mg Sodium

CHOICES: 1/2 Grains & Starches; 1/2 Fruits; 2 Meat & Alternatives; 1 Fats

Mango Jicama Scallops

Scallops cook so quickly on the grill that you'll be rewarded with an upscale, impressive dinner in less time than it takes to make reservations! Make the salsa first and let it stand to blend the flavours while you grill the scallops.

JICAMA SALSA

Chopped frozen mango pieces, thawed	1 cup	250 mL
Grated peeled jicama	1 cup	250 mL
Finely chopped red pepper	2 tbsp.	30 mL
Chopped fresh basil	1 tbsp.	15 mL
Lime juice	1 tbsp.	15 mL
Sliced green onion	1 tbsp.	15 mL
Brown sugar, packed	1 tsp.	5 mL
Finely grated gingerroot	1 tsp.	5 mL
Cayenne pepper, just a pinch		

SCALLOPS

Large sea scallops	1 lb.	454 g
Bamboo skewers (8 inches, 20 cm, each), soaked in water for 10 minutes	8	8
Canola oil	1 tsp.	5 mL
Salt, sprinkle		
Pepper, sprinkle		

Jicama Salsa: Preheat gas barbecue to medium-high (see Tip, page 77). Combine all 9 ingredients in small bowl. Let stand for 30 minutes to blend flavours. Makes about 2 cups (500 mL) salsa.

Scallops: Thread scallops onto skewers (see Note). Brush with canola oil. Sprinkle with salt and pepper. Cook on greased grill for about 2 minutes per side until opaque. Serve with Jicama Salsa. Serves 4.

1 serving: 156 Calories; 2.2 g Total Fat (0.8 g Mono, 0.7 g Poly, 0.2 g Sat); 37 mg Cholesterol; 14 g Carbohydrate; 2 g Fibre; 20 g Protein; 185 mg Sodium

CHOICES: 1/2 Fruits; 2 1/2 Meat & Alternatives

Pictured on page 107.

Note: Use 2 skewers for each scallop skewer for better control when turning on grill.

Jalapeño Halibut

Try this tangy, spicy substitute for high-fat tartar sauce tonight—just for the halibut!

Halibut fillets, any small bones removed (about 4 – 5 oz., 113 – 140 g, each)	4	4
Salt	1/4 tsp.	1 mL
Pepper	1/4 tsp.	1 mL
Light creamy Caesar dressing	2 tbsp.	30 mL
Light mayonnaise	1 tbsp.	15 mL
Finely chopped pickled jalapeño pepper (see Tip, page 130)	1 tsp.	5 mL

Preheat oven to 425°F (220°C). Arrange fillets on greased baking sheet. Sprinkle with salt and pepper.

Combine remaining 3 ingredients in small cup. Spread over fillets. Bake for about 7 minutes until fish flakes easily when tested with fork. Serves 4.

1 serving: 146 Calories; 4.2 g Total Fat (1.6 g Mono, 1.4 g Poly, 0.4 g Sat); 38 mg Cholesterol; 2 g Carbohydrate; trace Fibre; 24 g Protein; 330 mg Sodium

CHOICES: 3 Meat & Alternatives

Saucy Seafood Grill

Your barbecue can do more than just grill! Here, it gently cooks delicate seafood in a sweet and spicy chili sauce. Any extra sauce goes great over pasta, rice or veggies.

Sweet chili sauce	1/3 cup	75 mL
Low-sodium soy sauce	2 tbsp.	30 mL
Chili paste (sambal oelek)	1/2 tsp.	2 mL
Small bay scallops	3/4 lb.	340 g
Uncooked medium shrimp (peeled and deveined)	3/4 lb.	340 g
Haddock fillet, cut into 1 inch (2.5 cm) pieces	1/2 lb.	225 g

(continued on next page)

Fish & Seafood

Preheat gas barbecue to medium-high. Combine first 3 ingredients in medium bowl.

Add remaining 3 ingredients. Stir until coated. Transfer to 2 greased 9 inch (22 cm) foil pie plates. Cover with foil. Place on grill. Cook for about 6 minutes, stirring once, until scallops are opaque, shrimp turn pink and fish flakes easily when tested with fork. Makes about 5 cups (1.25 L). Serves 6.

1 serving: 169 Calories; 1.7 g Total Fat (0.2 g Mono, 0.6 g Poly, 0.3 g Sat); 126 mg Cholesterol; 8 g Carbohydrate; trace Fibre; 28 g Protein; 498 mg Sodium

CHOICES: 4 Meat & Alternatives

Saucy Shrimp And Fennel

Cook gourmet the easy way—in your microwave! This hearty combination makes lots of sauce to spoon over rice or pasta.

Chunky tomato pasta sauce	2 cups	500 mL
Thinly sliced fennel bulb (white part only)	2 cups	500 mL
Thinly sliced celery	1 cup	250 mL
Prepared vegetable broth	1/4 cup	60 mL
Pepper	1/4 tsp.	1 mL
Cooked medium shrimp (peeled and deveined)	3/4 lb.	340 g

Combine first 5 ingredients in 2 quart (2 L) casserole. Microwave, covered, on high (100%) for about 13 minutes, stirring every 3 minutes, until fennel starts to soften.

Add shrimp. Stir. Microwave, covered, on high (100%) for about 2 minutes until shrimp are heated through. Makes about 5 cups (1.25 L). Serves 4.

1 serving: 198 Calories; 1.9 g Total Fat (0.2 g Mono, 0.4 g Poly, 0.3 g Sat); 166 mg Cholesterol; 27 g Carbohydrate; 6 g Fibre; 22 g Protein; 660 mg Sodium

CHOICES: 4 Vegetables; 2 Meat & Alternatives

Thai Haddock Stir-Fry

This family-friendly stir-fry won't "Thai" you up in the kitchen for long!
Super-speedy to make and best served with brown rice.

Canola oil	2 tsp.	10 mL
Haddock fillets, any small bones removed, cut into 1 inch (2.5 cm) pieces	1 lb.	454 g
Prepared vegetable broth	1 cup	250 mL
Brown sugar, packed	1 tbsp.	15 mL
Lime juice	1 tbsp.	15 mL
Garlic powder	1/2 tsp.	2 mL
Ground ginger	1/2 tsp.	2 mL
Thai red curry paste	1/2 tsp.	2 mL
Frozen Oriental mixed vegetables	6 cups	1.5 L
Soy sauce	1 tbsp.	15 mL
Cornstarch	1 tbsp.	15 mL

Heat wok or large frying pan on medium-high until very hot. Add cooking oil. Add fish. Stir-fry for 2 to 3 minutes until fish flakes easily when tested with fork. Remove to small bowl with slotted spoon. Cover to keep warm.

Add next 6 ingredients to same frying pan. Stir. Bring to a boil. Add vegetables. Cook, covered, for about 3 minutes, stirring occasionally, until tender-crisp.

Stir soy sauce into cornstarch in small cup. Add to vegetable mixture. Heat and stir for about 1 minute until boiling and thickened. Add fish. Stir gently. Makes about 4 1/2 cups (1.1 L). Serves 4.

1 serving: 210 Calories; 3.4 g Total Fat (1.5 g Mono, 1.0 g Poly, 0.4 g Sat); 65 mg Cholesterol; 19 g Carbohydrate; 5 g Fibre; 24 g Protein; 482 mg Sodium

CHOICES: 1 Vegetables; 3 Meat & Alternatives

Paré Pointer

Dragons sleep all day because they hunt knights.

Cajun-Stuffed Trout

For an impressive dinner, you can't beat a stuffed fish—and you won't believe
how quick and easy it is to make! These trout are filled with
mildly spiced rice and vegetables.

Whole rainbow trout (7 – 8 oz., 200 – 225 g, each), pan-ready	2	2
Cajun seasoning	1/4 tsp.	1 mL
Canola oil	1 tsp.	5 mL
Chopped onion	1/4 cup	60 mL
Chopped red pepper	1/4 cup	60 mL
Cajun seasoning	1 tsp.	5 mL
Cooked converted rice (about 3 tbsp., 50 mL, uncooked)	1/2 cup	125 mL
Fat-free ranch dressing	1 tbsp.	15 mL

Preheat oven to 400°F (205°C). Sprinkle half of first amount of seasoning inside each fish.

Heat canola oil in small frying pan on medium. Add next 3 ingredients. Cook for about 2 minutes, stirring often, until onion starts to soften.

Add rice. Heat and stir for 1 minute. Remove from heat.

Add dressing. Stir well. Place fish on greased baking sheet. Spoon rice mixture into fish. Spread evenly. Bake for 10 to 12 minutes until fish flakes easily when tested with fork. Serves 4.

1 serving: 205 Calories; 7.1 g Total Fat (2.4 g Mono, 2.2 g Poly, 1.7 g Sat); 69 mg Cholesterol;
10 g Carbohydrate; trace Fibre; 24 g Protein; 269 mg Sodium

CHOICES: 1/2 Grains & Starches; 3 Meat & Alternatives

Scallop And Asparagus Rotini

Asparagus, scallops, and lemon make for one dynamite combination! A sprinkling of fresh dill rounds out the flavour perfectly.

Water	8 cups	2 L
Salt	1 tsp.	5 mL
Whole-wheat rotini	8 oz.	225 g
Canola oil	1 tsp.	5 mL
Fresh asparagus, trimmed of tough ends, cut into 2 inch (5 cm) pieces	1 lb.	454 g
Garlic cloves, minced (or 1/2 tsp., 2 mL, powder)	2	2
Prepared vegetable broth	1 cup	250 mL
Salt	1/2 tsp.	2 mL
Pepper	1/4 tsp.	1 mL
Prepared vegetable broth	2 tbsp.	30 mL
Cornstarch	1 tbsp.	15 mL
Small bay scallops	3/4 lb.	340 g
Lemon juice	2 tbsp.	30 mL
Chopped fresh dill (or 3/4 tsp., 4 mL, dried)	1 tbsp.	15 mL

Combine water and salt in large saucepan. Bring to a boil. Add pasta. Boil, uncovered, for 7 to 9 minutes, stirring occasionally, until tender but firm. Drain. Return to same pot. Cover to keep warm.

Heat wok or large frying pan on medium-high until very hot. Add canola oil. Add asparagus and garlic. Stir-fry for about 1 minute until garlic is fragrant. Add next 3 ingredients. Bring to a boil, stirring occasionally. Reduce heat to medium. Boil gently, uncovered, for about 3 minutes until asparagus starts to soften.

Stir second amount of broth into cornstarch in small cup. Add asparagus mixture to pan. Heat and stir for 1 minute until bubbling and thickened.

Add scallops. Stir. Cook for about 2 minutes, stirring often, until scallops turn opaque.

(continued on next page)

Add lemon juice and dill. Add to pasta. Stir. Makes about 6 cups (1.5 L). Serves 4.

1 serving: 344 Calories; 5.4 g Total Fat (0.7 g Mono, 0.6 g Poly, 0.7 g Sat); 28 mg Cholesterol; 47 g Carbohydrate; 11 g Fibre; 26 g Protein; 574 mg Sodium

CHOICES: 2 Grains & Starches; 2 Meat & Alternatives

Pictured on page 108.

Mustard Shrimp And Leek

Mustard's not just for hotdogs or sandwiches anymore! This spicy condiment adds heat and flavour to a medley of shrimp and leek.

Dijon mustard (with whole seeds)	1/4 cup	60 mL
White wine vinegar	1/4 cup	60 mL
Olive (or canola) oil	1 tbsp.	15 mL
Granulated sugar	1 tsp.	5 mL
Olive (or canola) oil	2 tsp.	10 mL
Sliced leek (white part only)	4 cups	1 L
Garlic clove, minced (or 1/4 tsp., 1 mL, powder)	1	1
Uncooked medium shrimp (peeled and deveined)	1 1/2 lbs.	680 g

Combine first 4 ingredients in small bowl. Set aside.

Heat second amount of olive oil in large frying pan on medium. Add leek and garlic. Cook for about 8 minutes, stirring occasionally, until softened.

Add shrimp and mustard mixture. Stir. Cook, covered, for about 5 minutes until shrimp turn pink. Makes about 6 cups (1.5 L). Serves 4.

1 serving: 318 Calories; 10.0 g Total Fat (4.6 g Mono, 1.8 g Poly, 1.4 g Sat); 259 mg Cholesterol; 20 g Carbohydrate; 3 g Fibre; 37 g Protein; 580 mg Sodium

CHOICES: 2 Vegetables: 5 Meat & Alternatives; 1 Fats

Tuscan Sole

Delicate, crumb-crusted fish fillets are served with a flavourful medley of roasted vegetables. This dish has definitely got sole!

TUSCAN VEGETABLES

Chopped zucchini (with peel), 1/2 inch (12 mm) pieces	2 cups	500 mL
Chopped onion	1 cup	250 mL
Grape tomatoes	24	24
Chopped fresh white mushrooms	1 cup	250 mL
Italian seasoning	2 tsp.	10 mL
Olive (or canola) oil	2 tsp.	10 mL
Pepper	1/4 tsp.	1 mL

CRUMB-TOPPED SOLE

Sole fillets (about 2 oz., 57 g, each), any small bones removed	8	8
Lemon juice	4 tsp.	20 mL
Crushed multigrain crackers	1/2 cup	125 mL

Tuscan Vegetables: Set oven racks on bottom and upper positions (see Note 1). Preheat oven to 475°F (240°C). Combine first 7 ingredients in large bowl. Toss until coated. Arrange in single layer on greased baking sheet with sides. Bake on lower rack for about 16 minutes, stirring at halftime, until vegetables start to brown. Makes about 3 cups (750 mL).

Crumb-Topped Sole: Meanwhile, arrange fillets on separate greased baking sheet (see Note 2). Sprinkle with lemon juice. Press 1 tbsp. (15 mL) cracker crumbs evenly on top of each fillet. Bake on upper rack for about 8 minutes until crumbs are golden and fish flakes easily when tested with fork. Serve with Tuscan Vegetables. Serves 4.

1 serving: 271 Calories; 6.4 g Total Fat (2.0 g Mono, 0.8 g Poly, 0.7 g Sat); 54 mg Cholesterol; 27 g Carbohydrate; 4 g Fibre; 25 g Protein; 349 mg Sodium

CHOICES: 1 Grains & Starches; 1 Vegetables; 3 Meat & Alternatives

Note 1: Upper rack is the position second from the top (about 7 inches, 18 cm, from element) in oven.

Note 2: Sole comes in various sizes and the tail end is usually thinner than the middle. To ensure even cooking, fold the thinner tail portion underneath and group smaller fillets together to create portions of uniform size and thickness.

Chili Ginger Salmon

Kick your taste buds into overdrive with chili and ginger, then cool them down with a burst of fresh lime. Serve with a side of colourful stir-fried or steamed veggies.

Sweet chili sauce	3 tbsp.	50 mL
Lime juice	1 tbsp.	15 mL
Finely grated gingerroot (or 1/4 tsp., 1 mL, ground ginger)	1 tsp.	5 mL
Salt, just a pinch		
Salmon fillets (4 – 5 oz., 113 – 140 g, each), skin removed	4	4
Chopped fresh basil	4 tsp.	20 mL
Lime wedges	4	4

Preheat broiler. Combine first 4 ingredients in small bowl.

Arrange salmon on baking sheet, lined with greased foil. Brush with chili sauce mixture. Broil on top rack in oven for about 5 minutes until fish flakes easily when tested with fork. Transfer to serving plate.

Sprinkle with basil. Serve with lime wedges. Serves 4.

1 serving: 226 Calories; 11.9 g Total Fat (5.1 g Mono, 2.4 g Poly, 2.8 g Sat); 75 mg Cholesterol; 5 g Carbohydrate; trace Fibre; 23 g Protein; 166 mg Sodium

CHOICES: 3 Meat & Alternatives

Pictured on page 107.

Paré Pointer
*You don't need training to be a garbage collector—
you just pick it up as you go along.*

Lime Hazelnut Tilapia

Spicy, nutty and citrusy flavours mingle in these crunchy hazelnut-crusted fillets. The light homemade tartar sauce makes for the perfect accompaniment.

All-purpose flour	1/4 cup	60 mL
Large egg, fork-beaten	1	1
Lime juice	1 tbsp.	15 mL
Tex Mex seasoning	1 tbsp.	15 mL
Grated lime zest	1 tsp.	5 mL
Fine dry bread crumbs	1/4 cup	60 mL
Chopped sliced hazelnuts (filberts)	1/3 cup	75 mL
Tilapia fillets (about 4 – 5 oz., 113 – 140 g, each), any small bones removed	4	4
TARTAR SAUCE		
Light mayonnaise	1/3 cup	75 mL
Chopped green onion	1 tbsp.	15 mL
Tangy dill relish	1 tbsp.	15 mL
Grated lime zest	1/2 tsp.	2 mL

Preheat oven to 425°F (220°C). Measure flour onto plate.

Combine next 4 ingredients in large shallow dish.

Combine bread crumbs and hazelnuts in small cup. Transfer to separate plate.

Press both sides of fillets into flour. Dip into egg mixture. Press both sides of fillets into crumb mixture until coated. Discard any remaining flour, egg mixture and bread crumb mixture. Arrange fillets on greased baking sheet. Bake for about 10 minutes until fish flakes easily when tested with fork.

Tartar Sauce: Combine all 4 ingredients in small bowl. Makes about 6 tbsp. (100 mL) sauce. Serve with fillets. Serves 4.

1 serving: 308 Calories; 16.3 g Total Fat (9.0 g Mono, 3.5 g Poly, 1.5 g Sat); 110 mg Cholesterol; 15 g Carbohydrate; 1 g Fibre; 27 g Protein; 430 mg Sodium

CHOICES: 1/2 Grains & Starches; 3 1/2 Meats & Alternatives; 2 Fats

Kaleidoscope Shrimp

A kaleidoscope of colours and flavours in this dish of fresh vegetables and shrimp, coated with a light lemon sauce and packed with peppery punch. Serve with brown basmati rice to sneak in a little extra fibre.

Prepared vegetable broth	1/3 cup	75 mL
Lemon juice	1/4 cup	60 mL
Sweet chili sauce	2 tbsp.	30 mL
Cornstarch	2 tsp.	10 mL
Coarsely ground pepper	1 tsp.	5 mL
Grated lemon zest	1/2 tsp.	2 mL
Canola oil	1 tbsp.	15 mL
Sugar snap peas, trimmed	2 cups	500 mL
Thinly sliced red pepper	2 cups	500 mL
Thinly sliced orange pepper	2 cups	500 mL
Can of cut baby corn, drained	14 oz.	398 mL
Thinly sliced red onion	1 cup	250 mL
Garlic cloves, minced	2	2
(or 1/2 tsp., 2 mL, powder)		
Uncooked large shrimp	1 lb.	454 g
(peeled and deveined)		

Combine first 6 ingredients in small cup. Set aside.

Heat wok or large frying pan on medium-high until very hot. Add canola oil. Add next 6 ingredients. Stir-fry for about 3 minutes until peppers start to soften.

Add shrimp. Stir-fry for about 3 minutes until shrimp turn pink. Stir broth mixture. Add to shrimp mixture. Heat and stir for about 1 minute until boiling and thickened. Makes about 7 cups (1.75 L). Serves 6.

1 serving: 264 Calories; 4.8 g Total Fat (1.8 g Mono, 1.7 g Poly, 0.6 g Sat); 115 mg Cholesterol; 37 g Carbohydrate; 6 g Fibre; 21 g Protein; 208 mg Sodium

CHOICES: 1 Grains & Starches; 2 Vegetables; 2 Meat & Alternatives; 1/2 Fats

Pictured on page 107.

Warm Mango Salsa Salmon

Don't just spoon cold salsa over salmon—warm your homemade salsa with the fish so the flavours can mingle. A quick and tasty dinner!

Diced frozen mango pieces	1 cup	250 mL
Diced kiwifruit	1/2 cup	125 mL
Finely chopped fresh jalapeño pepper (see Tip, page 130)	2 tbsp.	30 mL
Finely chopped red onion	2 tbsp.	30 mL
Lemon juice	1 tbsp.	15 mL
Lime juice	1 tbsp.	15 mL
Salt	1/2 tsp.	2 mL
Salmon fillets, skin removed, cut into 1 inch (2.5 cm) pieces	1 1/4 lbs.	560 g
Tub margarine	4 tsp.	20 mL
Light mayonnaise	2 tbsp.	30 mL
Chopped fresh parsley	1 tbsp.	15 mL

Preheat oven to 425°F (220°C). Combine first 7 ingredients in large bowl. Add salmon. Toss. Spread evenly in greased 9 x 13 inch (22 x 33 cm) baking dish.

Spoon margarine, in 1/2 tsp. (2 mL) amounts, over salmon mixture. Bake, uncovered, for about 12 minutes until fish flakes easily when tested with fork.

Add mayonnaise and parsley. Stir gently. Makes about 4 1/2 cups (1.1 L). Serves 4.

1 serving: 360 Calories; 21.4 g Total Fat (9.3 g Mono, 5.3 g Poly, 4.1 g Sat); 96 mg Cholesterol; 13 g Carbohydrate; 2 g Fibre; 29 g Protein; 475 mg Sodium

CHOICES: 1/2 Fruits; 4 Meat & Alternatives; 1 Fats

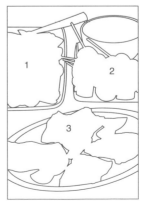

1. Kaleidoscope Shrimp, page 105
2. Mango Jicama Scallops, page 95
3. Chili Ginger Salmon, page 103

Props courtesy of: Casa Bugatti
Danesco Inc.

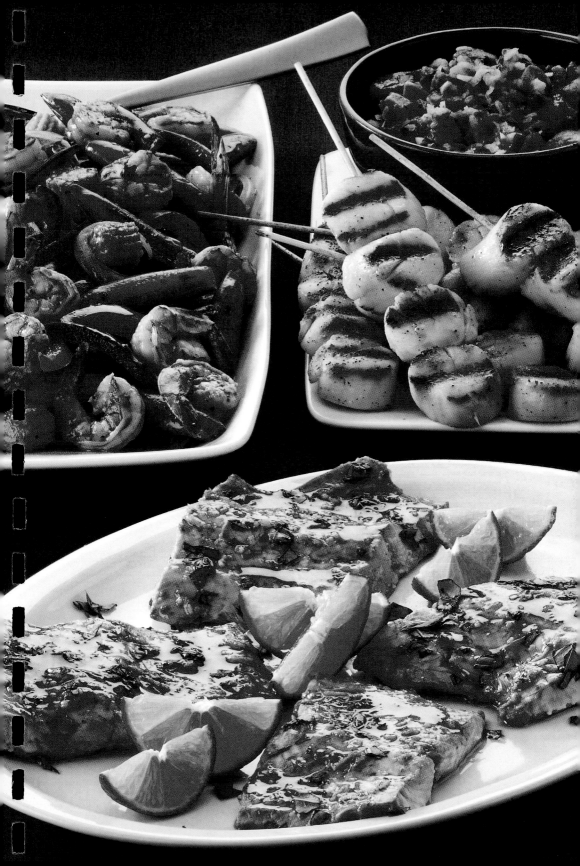

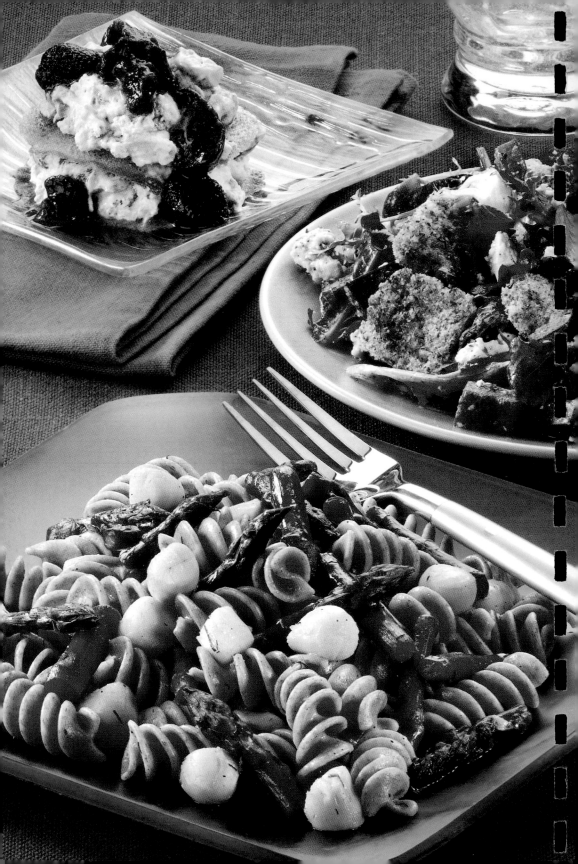

Mexican-Spiced Halibut

This incredibly easy dish, enlivened with the flavours of Mexico, packs a
punch that will send your taste buds south of the border. Olè!

Olive (or canola) oil	1 1/2 tbsp.	25 mL
Paprika	1 tbsp.	15 mL
Dried oregano	1 1/2 tsp.	7 mL
Grated lime zest	1/2 tsp.	2 mL
Ground cumin	1/2 tsp.	2 mL
Dried crushed chilies	1/4 tsp.	1 mL
Salt	1/4 tsp.	1 mL
Pepper	1/2 tsp.	2 mL
Halibut fillets (about 4 – 5 oz., 113 – 140 g, each), any small bones removed	4	4

Preheat broiler. Combine first 8 ingredients in small bowl.

Rub fillets with spice mixture. Place on greased baking sheet. Broil on top
rack in oven for about 5 minutes until fish flakes easily when tested with
fork. Serves 4.

1 serving: 178 Calories; 8.0 g Total Fat (4.6 g Mono, 1.4 g Poly, 1.1 g Sat); 36 mg Cholesterol;
2 g Carbohydrate; 1 g Fibre; 24 g Protein; 209 mg Sodium

CHOICES: 3 Meat & Alternatives; 1 Fats

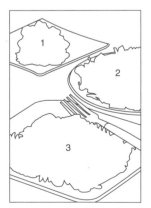

1. Strawberry Wafer Layers, page 148
2. Greek Bread Salad, page 31
3. Scallop And Asparagus Rotini, page 100

Props courtesy of: Danesco Inc.

Santa Fe Salmon Stew

This saucy stew is full of salmon and potatoes with just a hint of heat. Enjoy with a slice of crusty whole-wheat bread to soak up the delicious sauce.

Small red baby potatoes, cut in half	3/4 lb.	340 g
Canola oil	1 tsp.	5 mL
Chopped onion	1 cup	250 mL
Chopped celery	1/2 cup	125 mL
Canned black beans, rinsed and drained	1 cup	250 mL
Frozen kernel corn	1 cup	250 mL
Grated carrot	1/2 cup	125 mL
Can of diced green chilies	4 oz.	113 g
Chili powder	1 tsp.	5 mL
Finely chopped chipotle pepper in adobo sauce (see Tip, page 40)	1 tsp.	5 mL
Salt	1/4 tsp.	1 mL
All-purpose flour	2 tbsp.	30 mL
Prepared vegetable broth	2 cups	500 mL
Salmon fillets, skin removed, cut into 1 inch (2.5 cm) cubes	1 lb.	454 g
Skim evaporated milk	1/2 cup	125 mL

Put potatoes into medium microwave-safe bowl. Microwave, covered, on high (100%) for about 4 minutes until almost tender. Cover to keep warm.

Meanwhile, heat canola oil in large saucepan on medium-high. Add onion and celery. Cook, uncovered, for about 2 minutes, stirring often, until starting to soften.

Add next 7 ingredients. Stir. Cook, uncovered, for about 2 minutes, stirring occasionally, until fragrant.

Add flour. Heat and stir for 1 minute. Slowly add broth, stirring constantly, until boiling and thickened.

Add salmon, evaporated milk and potatoes. Stir. Bring to a boil. Reduce heat to medium-low. Simmer, covered, for about 5 minutes until fish flakes easily when tested with fork and potatoes are tender. Makes about 8 cups (2 L). Serves 4.

(continued on next page)

1 serving: 434 Calories; 13.7 g Total Fat (5.8 g Mono, 2.8 g Poly, 3.0 g Sat); 76 mg Cholesterol; 46 g Carbohydrate; 7 g Fibre; 32 g Protein; 802 mg Sodium

CHOICES: 2 Grains & Starches; 1 Vegetables; 3 1/2 Meat & Alternatives

---

Grilled Salmon With Ginger Cream

Fresh and flavourful! A simple, satisfying supper of fresh salmon, dressed up in a pretty pink and green-speckled sauce.

Salmon fillets (4 – 5 oz., 113 – 140 g, each), skin removed	4	4
Olive (or canola) oil	2 tsp.	10 mL
Salt, sprinkle		
Pepper, sprinkle		
GINGER CREAM		
Light mayonnaise	1/4 cup	60 mL
Light sour cream	1/4 cup	60 mL
Finely chopped celery	2 tbsp.	30 mL
Chopped fresh parsley	1 tbsp.	15 mL
Finely chopped pickled ginger slices	1 tbsp.	15 mL
Sliced green onion	1 tbsp.	15 mL

Preheat gas barbecue to medium. Brush salmon with olive oil. Sprinkle with salt and pepper. Cook on greased grill for about 2 minutes per side until fish flakes easily when tested with fork.

Ginger Cream: Combine all 6 ingredients in small bowl. Serve with salmon. Serves 4.

1 serving: 300 Calories; 20.4 g Total Fat (9.2 g Mono, 4.1 g Poly, 3.9 g Sat); 85 mg Cholesterol; 4 g Carbohydrate; trace Fibre; 24 g Protein; 217 mg Sodium

CHOICES: 3 Meat & Alternatives; 1 1/2 Fats

Mixed-Bean Tagine

Although a tagine is traditionally simmered for a long period of time, this meatless version cooks up tangy and tasty in less than 30 minutes. Serve this saucy stew of tomato and beans over couscous, rice or pasta.

Canola oil	2 tsp.	10 mL
Chopped celery	1 cup	250 mL
Chopped onion	1 cup	250 mL
Garlic cloves, minced	2	2
(or 1/2 tsp., 2 mL, powder)		
Ground ginger	1 tsp.	5 mL
Ground cumin	1/2 tsp.	2 mL
Ground cinnamon	1/4 tsp.	1 mL
Salt	1/4 tsp.	1 mL
Pepper	1/4 tsp.	1 mL
Can of diced tomatoes (with juice)	28 oz.	796 mL
Can of mixed beans, rinsed and drained	19 oz.	540 mL
Liquid honey	1 tbsp.	15 mL
Lemon juice	2 tsp.	10 mL

Heat canola oil in large saucepan on medium. Add next 8 ingredients. Cook, uncovered, for about 5 minutes, stirring often, until onion is softened.

Add remaining 4 ingredients. Stir. Bring to a boil. Boil gently, partially covered, for 5 minutes to blend flavours. Makes about 5 1/2 cups (1.4 L). Serves 4.

1 serving: 201 Calories; 3.0 g Total Fat (1.4 g Mono, 0.7 g Poly, 0.2 g Sat); 0 mg Cholesterol; 38 g Carbohydrate; 6 g Fibre; 10 g Protein; 869 mg Sodium

CHOICES: 1 Grains & Starches; 2 Vegetables; 1 Meat & Alternatives

Pictured on page 126.

Edamame Curry Bowl

Edamame, cauliflower and sweet potato are tossed in a flavourful and spicy sauce. Serve with pasta or rice.

Canola oil	1 tsp.	5 mL
Cauliflower florets	2 cups	500 mL
Chopped onion	1 cup	250 mL
Brown sugar, packed	1 tsp.	5 mL
Thai red curry paste	1/2 tsp.	2 mL
Salt	1/2 tsp.	2 mL
Pepper	1/4 tsp.	1 mL
Prepared vegetable broth	2 cups	500 mL
Frozen shelled edamame (soybeans)	1 1/2 cups	375 mL
Garlic cloves, minced	2	2
(or 1/2 tsp., 2 mL, powder)		
Can of sweet potatoes, drained	19 oz.	540 mL
and chopped		
Prepared vegetable broth	1 tbsp.	15 mL
Cornstarch	1 tbsp.	15 mL

Heat canola oil in large frying pan on medium-high. Add next 6 ingredients. Cook for about 5 minutes, stirring often, until onion is softened.

Add next 3 ingredients. Stir. Bring to a boil. Reduce heat to medium. Cook, covered, for about 5 minutes until cauliflower is tender.

Add sweet potato. Stir second amount of broth into cornstarch in small cup. Add to cauliflower mixture. Heat and stir for about 2 minutes until sweet potato is heated through and sauce is boiling and thickened. Makes about 5 cups (1.25 L). Serves 4.

1 serving: 300 Calories; 5.0 g Total Fat (0.7 g Mono, 0.6 g Poly, 0.5 g Sat); 0 mg Cholesterol; 56 g Carbohydrate; 10 g Fibre; 11 g Protein; 646 mg Sodium

CHOICES: 2 1/2 Grains & Starches; 1 Vegetables

Orzo-Stuffed Peppers

Orzo for everyone! Keep the whole family happy when they each get their own portion of orzo, packed into tender-crisp red peppers with pecans, veggies and Parmesan cheese.

Diced zucchini (with peel)	1 cup	250 mL
Prepared vegetable broth	1 cup	250 mL
Chopped onion	1/2 cup	125 mL
Grated carrot	1/2 cup	125 mL
Orzo	1/2 cup	125 mL
Garlic and herb no-salt seasoning	1/2 tsp.	2 mL
Pepper	1/8 tsp.	0.5 mL
Chopped pecans, toasted (see Tip, below)	1/4 cup	60 mL
Grated light Parmesan cheese	2 tbsp.	30 mL
Water	2 tbsp.	30 mL
Large red peppers, halved lengthwise	2	2

Combine first 7 ingredients in medium microwave-safe bowl. Microwave, covered, on high (100%) for about 15 minutes, stirring every 5 minutes, until orzo is tender and liquid is absorbed.

Add pecans and cheese. Stir.

Pour water into greased 2 quart (2 L) casserole. Arrange pepper halves in casserole. Fill with orzo mixture. Microwave, covered, on high (100%) for about 5 minutes until peppers are tender-crisp. Makes 4 stuffed peppers.

1 stuffed pepper: 211 Calories; 6.6 g Total Fat (3.0 g Mono, 1.8 g Poly, 0.6 g Sat); 2 mg Cholesterol; 34 g Carbohydrate; 4 g Fibre; 7 g Protein; 167 mg Sodium

CHOICES: 1 1/2 Grains & Starches; 1 Vegetables; 1 Fats

 tip
When toasting nuts, seeds or coconut, cooking times will vary for each type of nut—so never toast them together. For small amounts, place ingredient in an ungreased frying pan. Heat on medium for 3 to 5 minutes, stirring often, until golden. For larger amounts, spread ingredient evenly in an ungreased shallow pan. Bake in a 350°F (175°C) oven for 5 to 10 minutes, stirring or shaking often, until golden.

Meatless

Quinoa Lentil Simmer

Cooking the veggies and spices separate from the quinoa allows for full-flavour impact. Combine the two to create one super-powered meatless main course!

Prepared vegetable broth	2 cups	500 mL
Quinoa, rinsed and drained	1 cup	250 mL
Canola oil	2 tsp.	10 mL
Sliced fresh white mushrooms	4 cups	1 L
Thai red curry paste	1/2 tsp.	2 mL
Frozen Oriental mixed vegetables	6 cups	1.5 L
Can of lentils, rinsed and drained	19 oz.	540 mL
Thai peanut sauce	1/3 cup	75 mL

Bring broth to a boil in large saucepan. Add quinoa. Stir. Reduce heat to medium. Boil gently, covered, for about 18 minutes, without stirring, until tender.

Meanwhile, heat canola oil in large frying pan on medium-high. Add mushrooms and curry paste. Cook for about 10 minutes, stirring often, until starting to brown.

Add remaining 3 ingredients. Stir. Cook, covered, for about 5 minutes until vegetables are heated through. Add quinoa. Stir. Makes about 9 1/2 cups (2.4 L). Serves 6.

1 serving: 278 Calories; 5.9 g Total Fat (1.3 g Mono, 1.1 g Poly, 0.8 g Sat); 0 mg Cholesterol; 44 g Carbohydrate; 12 g Fibre; 13 g Protein; 576 mg Sodium

CHOICES: 1 1/2 Grains & Starches; 1 Vegetables; 1 Meat & Alternatives

Pictured on page 126.

Chickpea Spinach Fajitas

Looking for a quick lunch or dinner? These family-friendly fajitas will have you saying "that's a wrap!" in no time.

Canola oil	2 tsp.	10 mL
Sliced onion	1 cup	250 mL
Sliced red pepper	1 cup	250 mL
Garlic clove, minced (or 1/4 tsp., 1 mL, powder)	1	1
Ground cumin	1/2 tsp.	2 mL
Pepper	1/4 tsp.	1 mL
Can of chickpeas (garbanzo beans), rinsed and drained	19 oz.	540 mL
Fresh spinach leaves, lightly packed	2 cups	500 mL
Tomato sauce	1/2 cup	125 mL
Light sour cream	1/2 cup	125 mL
Whole wheat flour tortillas (9 inch, 22 cm, diameter)	4	4
Shredded lettuce, lightly packed	2 cups	500 mL
Diced tomato	1 cup	250 mL

Heat canola oil in large frying pan on medium-high. Add next 5 ingredients. Stir-fry for about 2 minutes until onion starts to soften.

Measure 1 cup (250 mL) chickpeas into small bowl. Mash. Add to onion mixture. Add spinach, tomato sauce and remaining chickpeas. Stir. Cook, covered, for about 2 minutes until spinach is wilted. Remove from heat.

Add sour cream. Stir.

Meanwhile, stack tortillas on work surface. Wrap in damp tea towel. Microwave on medium (50%) for about 2 minutes until warmed. Arrange tortillas on work surface. Scatter lettuce and tomato over top. Spoon chickpea mixture over tomato. Fold bottom end of each tortilla over filling. Fold in sides. Fold over from bottom to enclose filling. Makes 4 fajitas.

1 fajita: 322 Calories; 8.6 g Total Fat (1.9 g Mono, 3.0 g Poly, 1.8 g Sat); 10 mg Cholesterol; 51 g Carbohydrate; 10 g Fibre; 13 g Protein; 599 mg Sodium

CHOICES: 2 Grains & Starches; 1 1/2 Vegetables; 1/2 Meat & Alternatives; 1 Fats

Grilled Eggplant Parmigiana

Simple to prepare, yet elegant. This easy grilled casserole is a fun new twist on a hearty Italian classic. Everything is cooked on the grill, so you don't have to run back and forth between barbecue and stove.

Roasted garlic tomato pasta sauce	2 cups	500 mL
Chopped fresh parsley (or 1 1/2 tsp., 7 mL, flakes)	2 tbsp.	30 mL
Dried crushed chilies	1/4 tsp.	1 mL
Dried oregano	1/4 tsp.	1 mL
Pepper	1/4 tsp.	1 mL
Medium eggplants (with peel), cut crosswise into 8 slices each	2	2
Olive (or canola) oil	2 tbsp.	30 mL
Grated part-skim mozzarella cheese	2 cups	500 mL

Preheat gas barbecue to medium-high. Combine first 5 ingredients in medium saucepan. Place on 1 side of grill (see Note). Close lid. Cook, covered, for about 10 minutes, stirring occasionally, to blend flavours.

Meanwhile, brush both sides of eggplant slices with olive oil. Place on greased grill. Cook for about 3 minutes per side until tender. Arrange 8 slices of eggplant in bottom of greased 9 x 13 inch (22 x 33 cm) baking pan. Spoon half of sauce over eggplant. Spread evenly.

Sprinkle with half of cheese. Repeat with remaining eggplant slices, sauce and cheese. Place pan on grill. Close lid. Cook for about 5 minutes until sauce is bubbly and cheese is melted. Serves 4.

1 serving: 351 Calories; 18.7 g Total Fat (8.1 g Mono, 1.1 g Poly, 7.9 g Sat); 39 mg Cholesterol; 28 g Carbohydrate; 9 g Fibre; 21 g Protein; 645 mg Sodium

CHOICES: 3 Vegetables; 2 Meat & Alternatives; 1 Fats

Note: If your saucepan doesn't have a heatproof handle, wrap the handle in foil before placing on the grill and try to keep it away from any flames.

Greek Bulgur Burgers

Beef burgers have met their match! These meatless patties are filled with the fabulous flavours of peppers, spinach and oregano. Both delicious and nutritious.

Canola oil	1 tsp.	5 mL
Chopped onion	1 cup	250 mL
Chopped roasted red pepper	1 cup	250 mL
Greek seasoning	1 tsp.	5 mL
Dried oregano	1/2 tsp.	2 mL
Pepper	1/4 tsp.	1 mL
Prepared vegetable broth	3/4 cup	175 mL
Bulgur	1/2 cup	125 mL
Fresh spinach leaves, lightly packed, chopped	4 cups	1 L
Fine dry bread crumbs	2/3 cup	150 mL
Crumbled light feta cheese	1/2 cup	125 mL

Cooking spray

Preheat broiler. Heat canola oil in large frying pan on medium-high. Add next 5 ingredients. Cook for about 3 minutes, stirring often, until onion and red pepper are softened.

Add broth. Bring to a boil. Add bulgur. Boil, uncovered, for about 2 minutes until bulgur is tender and liquid is absorbed. Remove from heat.

Add spinach. Heat and stir for about 2 minutes until spinach starts to wilt. Transfer to large bowl.

Add bread crumbs and cheese. Stir. Measure 1/2 cup (125 mL) portions onto greased baking sheet. Shape into 1/2 inch (12 mm) thick patties.

Spray with cooking spray. Broil for about 10 minutes per side, turning at halftime, until browned. Makes 6 burgers.

1 burger: 167 Calories; 4.2 g Total Fat (0.8 g Mono, 0.5 g Poly, 1.6 g Sat); 7 mg Cholesterol; 26 g Carbohydrate; 4 g Fibre; 8 g Protein; 568 mg Sodium

CHOICES: 1 Grains & Starches; 1 Vegetables; 1/2 Meat & Alternatives

Spaghetti Squash 'N' Sauce

The most fun you'll ever have with a meatless dish! The pasta-like strands of spaghetti squash offer a truly unique presentation.

Small spaghetti squash (about 1 1/2 – 2 lbs., 680 – 900 g)	1	1
Olive oil	2 tsp.	10 mL
Sliced fresh white mushrooms	2 cups	500 mL
Garlic cloves, minced (or 1/2 tsp., 2 mL, powder)	2	2
Chopped onion	1/2 cup	125 mL
Chopped red pepper	1/2 cup	125 mL
Can of diced tomatoes (with juice)	14 oz.	398 mL
Dried thyme	1/2 tsp.	2 mL
Granulated sugar	1/2 tsp.	2 mL
Salt	1/4 tsp.	1 mL
Pepper	1/8 tsp	0.5 mL
Grated Parmesan cheese	2 tsp.	10 mL

Cut squash in half lengthwise. Remove seeds. Cut squash halves crosswise to make 4 pieces. Arrange in ungreased 3 quart (3 L) casserole. Microwave, covered, on high (100%) for about 15 minutes until squash strands separate easily when tested with fork. Cover to keep warm.

Meanwhile, heat olive oil in large frying pan on medium. Add next 4 ingredients. Cook for about 5 minutes, stirring often, until onion is softened.

Add next 5 ingredients. Cook and stir for 2 minutes to blend flavours.

Loosen squash strands with fork, leaving strands in shells. Spoon tomato mixture over top.

Sprinkle with cheese. Serves 4.

1 serving: 119 Calories; 3.7 g Total Fat (1.8 g Mono, 0.7 g Poly, 0.7 g Sat); 1 mg Cholesterol; 21 g Carbohydrate; 3 g Fibre; 3 g Protein; 469 mg Sodium

CHOICES: 3 Vegetables; 1/2 Fats

Zucchini Chickpea Toss

This hearty blend of roasted veggies has lots of protein from chickpeas, and plenty of flavour from cheese and sun-dried tomato pesto.

Chopped zucchini (with peel), 3/4 inch (2 cm) pieces	4 cups	1 L
Chopped green pepper	1 1/2 cups	375 mL
Chopped red pepper	1 1/2 cups	375 mL
Can of chickpeas (garbanzo beans), rinsed and drained	19 oz.	540 mL
Grated Romano cheese	2 tbsp.	30 mL
Sun-dried tomato pesto	1 tbsp.	15 mL
Red wine vinegar	2 tsp.	10 mL
Pepper	1/4 tsp.	1 mL

Preheat broiler. Arrange first 3 ingredients in single layer on ungreased baking sheet with sides. Broil on top rack in oven for 5 minutes. Stir. Broil for another 3 minutes until tender and starting to turn brown.

Meanwhile, put chickpeas into large microwave-safe bowl. Microwave, covered, on high (100%) for about 3 minutes until heated through. Add vegetables. Toss.

Add remaining 4 ingredients. Toss. Makes about 6 cups (1.5 L). Serves 4.

1 serving: 174 Calories; 3.4 g Total Fat (0.8 g Mono, 1.3 g Poly, 0.7 g Sat); 3 mg Cholesterol; 29 g Carbohydrate; 9 g Fibre; 10 g Protein; 237 mg Sodium

CHOICES: 1 Grains & Starches; 1 Vegetables; 1 Meat & Alternatives

 tip If a recipe calls for less than an entire can of tomato paste, freeze the unopened can for 30 minutes. Open both ends and push the contents through one end. Slice off only what you need. Freeze the remaining paste in a resealable freezer bag or plastic wrap for future use.

Mushroom Tofu Ragout

Tofu, the chameleon of the food world, absorbs the flavours of the ingredients it's cooked with—in this case, earthy mushrooms in a rich and savoury stew. Great served over pasta or with fresh bread.

Package of medium tofu, diced	1 lb.	454 g
Canola oil	1 tbsp.	15 mL
Sliced portobello mushrooms	4 cups	1 L
Sliced fresh white mushrooms	2 cups	500 mL
Chopped onion	1 1/2 cups	375 mL
Dried thyme	1/2 tsp.	2 mL
Paprika	1/2 tsp.	2 mL
Seasoned salt	1/2 tsp.	2 mL
Pepper	1/4 tsp.	1 mL
All-purpose flour	3 tbsp.	50 mL
Tomato paste (see Tip, page 120)	2 tbsp.	30 mL
Prepared vegetable broth	2 cups	500 mL
Light sour cream	3 tbsp.	50 mL
Chopped fresh parsley	2 tbsp.	30 mL
(or 1 1/2 tsp., 7 mL, flakes)		
Dijon mustard	1 tbsp.	15 mL

Put tofu on paper towel-lined plate to drain.

Heat canola oil in large saucepan or Dutch oven on medium-high. Add next 7 ingredients. Cook, uncovered, for about 5 minutes, stirring often, until onion is softened and mushrooms start to brown.

Add flour and tomato paste. Heat and stir for 1 minute. Slowly add vegetable broth, stirring constantly until boiling and thickened. Reduce heat to medium. Boil gently, uncovered, for 5 minutes to blend flavours. Add tofu. Stir. Boil gently, uncovered, for another 2 minutes, stirring occasionally, until heated through.

Add remaining 3 ingredients. Stir. Makes about 7 cups (1.75 L).

1 cup (250 mL): 120 Calories; 4.6 g Total Fat (1.5 g Mono, 1.6 g Poly, 0.8 g Sat); 2 mg Cholesterol; 13 g Carbohydrate; 2 g Fibre; 7 g Protein; 298 mg Sodium

CHOICES: 1 Vegetables; 1/2 Meat & Alternatives

Spicy Chickpea Bulgur

The subtle heat of this peppery bulgur is offset by sweet raisins and cashews.

Olive (or canola) oil	1 tsp.	5 mL
Chopped onion	1 cup	250 mL
Diced green pepper	1/2 cup	125 mL
Diced red pepper	1/2 cup	125 mL
Garlic cloves, minced	2	2
(or 1/2 tsp., 2 mL, powder)		
Chili powder	1 tsp.	5 mL
Dried crushed chilies	1/4 tsp.	1 mL
Ground cinnamon	1/4 tsp.	1 mL
Ground cumin	1/4 tsp.	1 mL
Salt	1/2 tsp.	2 mL
Pepper	1/4 tsp.	1 mL
Prepared vegetable broth	2 cups	500 mL
Can of chickpeas (garbanzo beans), rinsed and drained	19 oz.	540 mL
Bulgur	1 cup	250 mL
Dark raisins	1/2 cup	125 mL
Unsalted, roasted cashews	1/2 cup	125 mL
White vinegar	1 tbsp.	15 mL
Chopped fresh parsley	2 tsp.	10 mL

Heat olive oil in large frying pan on medium. Add next 10 ingredients. Cook for about 5 minutes, stirring often, until onion is softened.

Add broth. Bring to a boil, stirring occasionally. Add next 5 ingredients. Boil gently, uncovered, for about 5 minutes until bulgur is tender and liquid is absorbed.

Sprinkle with parsley. Makes about 6 cups (1.5 L). Serves 4.

1 serving: 451 Calories; 12.2 g Total Fat (6.1 g Mono, 2.8 g Poly, 1.9 g Sat); 0 mg Cholesterol; 77 g Carbohydrate; 13 g Fibre; 15 g Protein; 688 mg Sodium

CHOICES: 2 1/2 Grains & Starches; 1 Fruits; 1 Vegetables; 1 Meat & Alternatives; 2 Fats

Pictured on page 126.

Feta Creamed Spinach

Truly the crème de la crème *of spinach dishes. Here this leafy green is elevated to elegant fare with the addition of feta, mushrooms and back bacon.*

Tub margarine	1 1/2 tbsp.	25 mL
Chopped fresh white mushrooms	1 cup	250 mL
Garlic clove, minced	1	1
(or 1/4 tsp., 1 mL, powder)		
All-purpose flour	1 1/2 tbsp.	25 mL
Pepper, sprinkle		
Skim milk	1 cup	250 mL
Box of frozen chopped spinach,	10 oz.	300 g
thawed and squeezed dry		
Crumbled light feta cheese	1/2 cup	250 mL
Diced back (Canadian) bacon	1/4 cup	60 mL

Melt margarine in medium saucepan on medium. Add mushrooms and garlic. Cook, uncovered, for about 4 minutes, stirring occasionally, until liquid has evaporated.

Sprinkle with flour and pepper. Heat and stir for 1 minute. Slowly add milk, stirring constantly until boiling and thickened. Reduce heat to low.

Add remaining 3 ingredients. Cook, uncovered, for about 3 minutes, stirring occasionally, until heated through. Makes about 2 cups (500 mL). Serves 4.

1 serving: 157 Calories; 8.4 g Total Fat (2.2 g Mono, 1.9 g Poly, 3.0 g Sat); 16 mg Cholesterol; 10 g Carbohydrate; 2 g Fibre; 13 g Protein; 651 mg Sodium

CHOICES: 1 Meat & Alternatives; 1 Fats

Orange Veggie Medley

Add brightness and freshness to your next meal with this colourful and delicious medley of fresh vegetables in a sweet orange glaze.

Butternut squash, cut into 1/2 inch (12 mm) pieces	2 lbs.	900 g
Frozen peas	1 cup	250 mL
Chopped red pepper	1/2 cup	125 mL
Frozen concentrated orange juice, thawed	2 tbsp.	30 mL

Place squash in steamer basket. Place steamer basket in large saucepan. Pour boiling water into saucepan until within 1 inch (2.5 cm) of basket bottom. Cook, covered, on medium for about 7 minutes until squash is tender-crisp.

Add peas. Cook, covered, for about 3 minutes until peas are hot and squash is tender.

Combine red pepper and concentrated orange juice in large bowl. Add squash and peas. Toss. Makes about 4 cups (1 L). Serves 6.

1 serving: 99 Calories; 0.3 g Total Fat (trace Mono, 0.1 g Poly, 0.1 g Sat); 0 mg Cholesterol; 24 g Carbohydrate; 4 g Fibre; 3 g Protein; 33 mg Sodium

CHOICES: 3 Vegetables

Pictured on page 125.

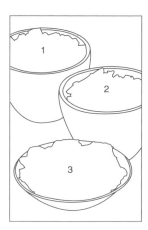

1. Orange Veggie Medley, above
2. Eat Your Greens, page 134
3. Lemon Oregano Vegetables, page 131

Props courtesy of: Danesco Inc.
· Totally Bamboo

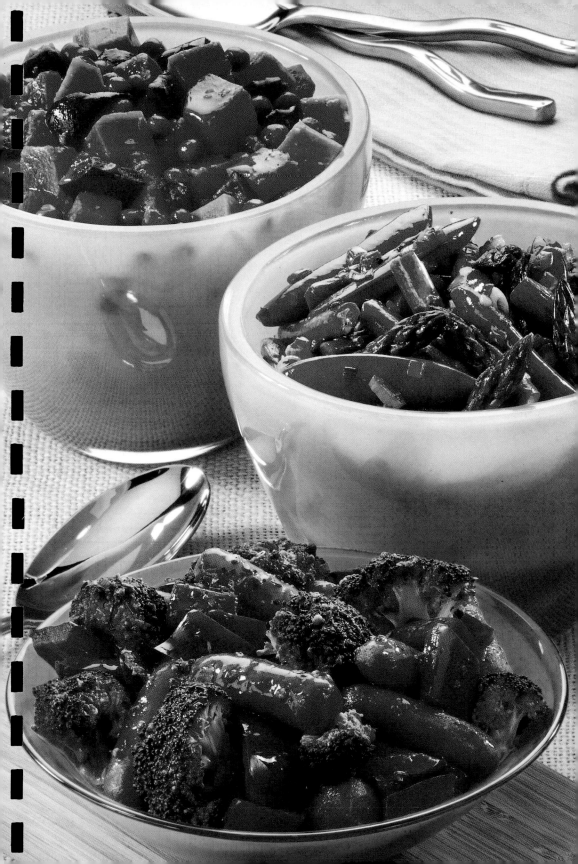

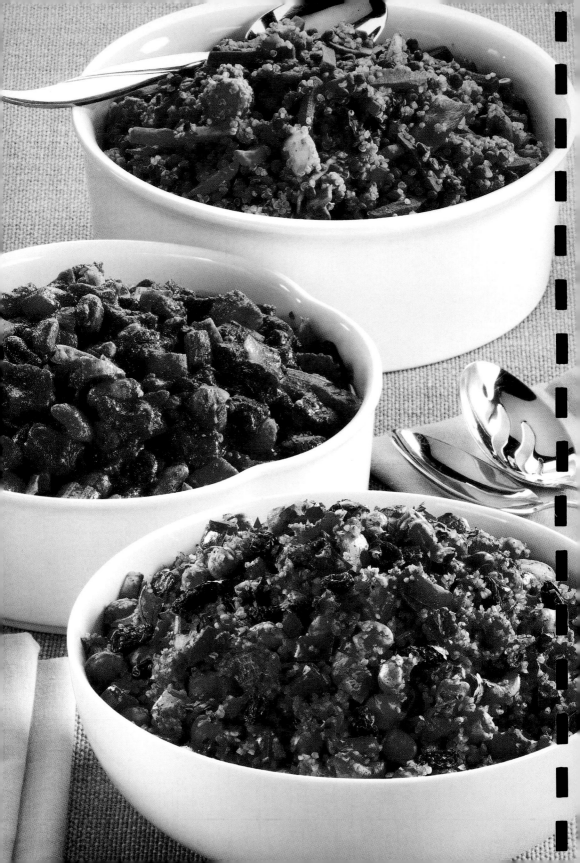

Oven-Roasted Parsnips

Roasting brings out a deliciously sweet, almost candy-like quality in parsnips.
An absolutely perfect side dish for a weekday supper, but classy
enough for company.

Large peeled parsnips, halved lengthwise and cut into 1/2 inch (12 mm) pieces (about 3 cups, 750 mL)	4	4
Water	2 tbsp.	30 mL
Canola oil	2 tbsp.	30 mL
Dried sage	1 tsp.	5 mL
Salt	1/4 tsp.	1 mL
Pepper	1/8 tsp.	0.5 mL

Preheat oven to 450°F (230°C). Put parsnip into large microwave-safe bowl. Sprinkle with water. Microwave, covered, on high (100%) for about 5 minutes until tender-crisp.

Add remaining 4 ingredients. Toss. Spread in single layer on greased baking sheet with sides. Bake for about 15 minutes, stirring twice, until tender and golden. Makes about 2 cups (500 mL). Serves 4.

1 serving: 136 Calories; 7.1 g Total Fat (4.1 g Mono, 2.1 g Poly, 0.6 g Sat); 0 mg Cholesterol; 18 g Carbohydrate; 3 g Fibre; 1 g Protein; 156 mg Sodium

CHOICES: 3 Vegetables; 1 Fats

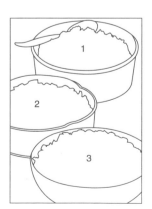

1. Quinoa Lentil Simmer, page 115
2. Mixed-Bean Tagine, page 112
3. Spicy Chickpea Bulgur, page 122

Props courtesy of: Pfaltzgraff Canada
Cherison Enterprises Inc.
The Bay

Roasted Broccoli

Why not bring out broccoli's naturally earthy flavour by roasting it? Add a drizzle of Dijon and garlic vinaigrette and you've got a very flavourful side.

Broccoli florets	5 cups	1.25 L
Canola oil	1 tbsp.	15 mL
Salt	1/4 tsp.	1 mL
Canola oil	1 tbsp.	15 mL
Red wine vinegar	1 tbsp.	15 mL
Dijon mustard	1/4 tsp.	1 mL
Garlic powder	1/4 tsp.	1 mL
Pepper	1/4 tsp.	1 mL

Preheat oven to 450°F (230°C). Put broccoli into large bowl. Drizzle with first amount of canola oil. Sprinkle with salt. Toss. Spread evenly on greased baking sheet with sides. Bake for about 15 minutes until browned and tender. Transfer to large serving bowl.

Meanwhile, combine remaining 5 ingredients in small cup. Drizzle over broccoli. Toss. Makes about 3 cups (750 mL). Serves 4.

1 serving: 86 Calories; 7.1 g Total Fat (4.0 g Mono, 2.2 g Poly, 0.5 g Sat); 0 mg Cholesterol; 5 g Carbohydrate; 3 g Fibre; 3 g Protein; 174 mg Sodium

CHOICES: 1 Fats

Broiled Tomatoes

Why mess with nature's perfection? Fresh, juicy tomatoes are at their finest when topped with a simple combination of cheese and onion.

Medium tomatoes	2	2
Finely chopped onion	2 tbsp.	30 mL
Grated Romano cheese	2 tbsp.	30 mL
Light mayonnaise	2 tbsp	30 mL

Preheat broiler. Cut tomatoes in half horizontally. Place, cut-side up, on ungreased baking sheet.

(continued on next page)

Combine next 3 ingredients in small bowl. Spread on tomatoes. Broil on centre rack in oven for about 4 minutes until cheese is golden and bubbly. Makes 4 tomatoes.

1 tomato: 57 Calories; 3.6 g Total Fat (1.5 g Mono, 0.8 g Poly, 0.5 g Sat); 6 mg Cholesterol; 5 g Carbohydrate; 1 g Fibre; 2 g Protein; 103 mg Sodium

CHOICES: 1/2 Vegetables; 1/2 Fats

Citrus Cauliflower

With fabulous flavour and a unique presentation that uses a whole head of cauliflower, it'll be easy to get your family to eat their vegetables!

Canola oil	2 tbsp.	30 mL
All-purpose flour	1 tbsp.	15 mL
Low-sodium prepared chicken broth	1/3 cup	75 mL
Milk	1/3 cup	75 mL
Lemon juice	1 tbsp.	15 mL
Grated lemon zest	1 tsp.	5 mL
Dried dillweed	1/4 tsp.	1 mL
Medium head of cauliflower, outer leaves trimmed (about 1 1/4 lbs., 560 g)	1	1
Low-sodium prepared chicken broth	1/4 cup	60 mL

Put canola oil into small microwave-safe bowl. Microwave, covered, on high (100%) for 15 seconds. Add flour. Stir until smooth. Add first amount of broth to flour mixture, stirring constantly, until smooth. Add milk. Stir. Microwave, covered, on medium (50%) for about 2 minutes, stirring every 45 seconds, until thickened.

Add next 3 ingredients. Stir. Cover to keep warm. Set aside.

Place cauliflower in deep 2 quart (2 L) casserole. Pour second amount of broth over top. Cover tightly. Microwave on high (100%) for about 8 minutes until tender-crisp. Pour sauce over cauliflower. Microwave, uncovered, on high (100%) for about 1 minute until heated through. Serves 4.

1 serving: 116 Calories; 7.0 g Total Fat (4.1 g Mono, 2.0 g Poly, 0.6 g Sat); 2 mg Cholesterol; 10 g Carbohydrate; 3 g Fibre; 4 g Protein; 143 mg Sodium

CHOICES: 1 Vegetables; 1 Fats

Couscous Mexicana

This colourful Mexican-inspired couscous is a fiesta for your taste buds.

Olive (or canola) oil	2 tsp.	10 mL
Chopped onion	1/2 cup	125 mL
Garlic clove, minced (or 1/4 tsp., 1 mL, powder)	1	1
Ground cumin	1/2 tsp.	2 mL
Prepared chicken broth	1 cup	250 mL
Couscous	3/4 cup	175 mL
Canned diced tomatoes, drained	1/2 cup	125 mL
Chopped green pepper	1/4 cup	60 mL
Chopped jalapeño pepper, seeds and ribs removed (see Tip, below)	2 tbsp.	30 mL
Chopped fresh cilantro	2 tbsp.	30 mL

Combine olive oil and onion in medium microwave-safe bowl. Microwave, covered, on high (100%) for about 2 minutes, stirring twice, until softened.

Add garlic and cumin. Stir. Microwave, covered, on high (100%) for about 1 minute until garlic is softened.

Add next 5 ingredients. Stir. Microwave, covered, on high (100%) for about 3 minutes, stirring occasionally, until couscous is tender and broth is absorbed.

Add cilantro. Stir. Makes about 3 cups (750 mL). Serves 6.

1 serving: 117 Calories; 1.9 g Total Fat (1.2 g Mono, 0.3 g Poly, 0.3 g Sat); 0 mg Cholesterol; 21 g Carbohydrate; 1 g Fibre; 4 g Protein; 299 mg Sodium

CHOICES: 1 Grains & Starches

 Hot peppers contain capsaicin in the seeds and ribs. Removing the seeds and ribs will reduce the heat. Wear rubber gloves when handling hot peppers and avoid touching your eyes. Wash your hands well afterwards.

Lemon Oregano Vegetables

What a smart idea! Use the cooking liquid from the vegetables to make a shiny lemon glaze. This helps to retain nutrients and flavour and adds some great visual appeal to these tasty, tender-crisp veggies.

Prepared chicken broth	1 cup	250 mL
Dried oregano	1 tsp.	5 mL
Baby carrots	1 cup	250 mL
Broccoli florets	1 cup	250 mL
Chopped red pepper	1 cup	250 mL
Lemon juice	1 tbsp.	30 mL
Cornstarch	1 tsp.	5 mL

Pepper, sprinkle

Combine broth and oregano in medium saucepan. Bring to a boil. Add carrots. Cook, uncovered, for about 5 minutes until starting to soften.

Add broccoli and red pepper. Reduce heat to medium. Cook, covered, for about 5 minutes until vegetables are tender-crisp. Remove to medium bowl with slotted spoon. Bring liquid to a boil.

Stir lemon juice into cornstarch in small cup. Add to boiling liquid. Heat and stir until thickened. Drizzle over vegetables.

Sprinkle with pepper. Toss. Makes about 2 1/2 cups (625 mL). Serves 4.

1 serving: 47 Calories; 0.8 g Total Fat (0.1 g Mono, 0.3 g Poly, 0.2 g Sat); 0 mg Cholesterol; 9 g Carbohydrate; 2 g Fibre; 2 g Protein; 397 mg Sodium

CHOICES: 1 Vegetables

Pictured on page 125.

Paré Pointer

Pulling a few strings will help you get ahead—especially if you're a puppeteer.

Cranberry Sweet Potatoes

Even though this combination of spice-scented sweet potatoes and tart cranberries has a holiday feel, you can serve it any time of year as a tasty, healthy side dish.

Tub margarine	1 tbsp.	15 mL
Diced onion	1 cup	250 mL
Cubed fresh peeled orange-fleshed sweet potato (about 1 lb., 454 g)	3 cups	750 mL
Frozen (or fresh) cranberries	1 cup	250 mL
Brown sugar, packed	3 tbsp.	50 mL
Orange juice	2 tbsp.	30 mL
Grated orange zest	1 tsp.	5 mL
Ground cinnamon	1/4 tsp.	1 mL
Ground ginger	1/4 tsp.	1 mL
Ground nutmeg	1/4 tsp.	1 mL
Salt	1/4 tsp.	1 mL

Melt margarine in 2 quart (2 L) casserole. Add onion. Stir. Microwave, covered, on high (100%) for about 3 minutes, stirring at halftime, until softened.

Add remaining 9 ingredients. Stir. Microwave, covered, on high (100%) for about 12 minutes, stirring twice, until sweet potato and cranberries are tender. Makes about 3 cups (750 mL). Serves 4.

1 serving: 184 Calories; 3.1 g Total Fat (1.2 g Mono, 1.2 g Poly, 0.5 g Sat); 0 mg Cholesterol; 38 g Carbohydrate; 5 g Fibre; 2 g Protein; 245 mg Sodium

CHOICES: 1 Grains & Starches; 1/2 Other Choices; 1/2 Fats

Paré Pointer

A grandfather clock is actually an old timer.

Potato Apple Cakes

Everyone loves potato cakes, but these have the added fresh flavour and goodness of apple.

Grated peeled baking potato	1 1/2 cups	375 mL
Grated peeled tart apple (such as Granny Smith)	1 cup	250 mL
Finely chopped celery	1/2 cup	125 mL
Chopped green onion	1/4 cup	60 mL
Seasoned salt	1 tsp.	5 mL
Grated lemon zest	1/2 tsp.	2 mL
Pepper	1/4 tsp.	1 mL
Large egg, fork-beaten	1	1
Whole-wheat flour	2 tbsp.	30 mL
Canola oil	2 tbsp.	30 mL

Squeeze potato and apple in paper towels to remove excess moisture. Put into medium bowl.

Add next 5 ingredients. Stir well.

Whisk egg and flour in small bowl until smooth. Add to potato mixture. Stir.

Meanwhile, heat 1 tbsp. (15 mL) canola oil in large frying pan on medium. Drop 4 portions of potato mixture, using about 1/4 cup (60 mL) for each, into pan. Flatten slightly. Cook for about 3 minutes per side until browned. Transfer to plate. Cover to keep warm. Repeat with remaining canola oil and potato mixture. Makes 8 cakes. Serves 4.

1 serving: 158 Calories; 11.8 g Total Fat (6.2 g Mono, 2.7 g Poly, 2.3 g Sat); 47 mg Cholesterol; 18 g Carbohydrate; 2 g Fibre; 3 g Protein; 396 mg Sodium

CHOICES: 1 Grains & Starches; 1 Fats

Eat Your Greens

You'd better believe your family will eat their greens when you dish up this tasty combination of crisp snap peas and asparagus.

Olive (or canola) oil	1 tbsp.	15 mL
Sliced green onion	1/2 cup	125 mL
Garlic clove, minced (or 1/4 tsp., 1 mL, powder)	1	1
Fresh asparagus, trimmed of tough ends, cut into 2 inch (5 cm) pieces	1 lb.	454 g
Sugar snap peas, trimmed	1 cup	250 mL
Low-sodium prepared chicken broth	1/4 cup	60 mL
Soy sauce	1 tsp.	5 mL
Coarsely ground pepper	1/2 tsp.	2 mL
Cornstarch	1/2 tsp.	2 mL

Heat olive oil in large frying pan on medium. Add green onion and garlic. Cook for about 2 minutes, stirring often, until onion is softened.

Add next 3 ingredients. Stir. Cook, covered, for about 3 minutes, stirring occasionally, until vegetables are tender-crisp.

Combine remaining 3 ingredients in small cup. Add to vegetables. Heat and stir until bubbling and vegetables are coated. Makes about 4 cups (1 L). Serves 6.

1 serving: 63 Calories; 2.3 g Total Fat (1.7 g Mono, 0.2 g Poly, 0.3 g Sat); trace Cholesterol; 7 g Carbohydrate; 3 g Fibre; 3 g Protein; 73 mg Sodium

CHOICES: 1 Vegetables; 1/2 Fats

Pictured on page 125.

Roasted Vegetable Quinoa

This light, flavourful Mediterranean-inspired side will have you yearning for the canals of Venice.

Water	1 1/2 cups	375 mL
Salt	1/8 tsp.	0.5 mL
Quinoa, rinsed and drained	1 cup	250 mL
Chopped red pepper	1 cup	250 mL
Chopped zucchini (with peel)	1 cup	250 mL
Chopped onion	1/2 cup	125 mL
Olive (or cooking) oil	2 tbsp.	30 mL
Dried rosemary, crushed	1/2 tsp.	2 mL
Salt	1/2 tsp.	2 mL
Pepper	1/4 tsp.	1 mL
Cherry tomatoes	10	10
Garlic clove, minced (or 1/4 tsp., 1 mL, powder)	1	1
Balsamic vinegar	3 tbsp.	50 mL
Liquid honey	2 tbsp.	30 mL
Olive (or canola) oil	1 tbsp.	15 mL

Preheat oven to 400°F (205°C). Combine water and salt in large saucepan. Bring to a boil. Add quinoa. Stir. Reduce heat to medium-low. Simmer, covered, for about 20 minutes, without stirring, until quinoa is tender and liquid is absorbed. Transfer to medium bowl. Fluff with fork. Cover to keep warm.

Meanwhile, put next 3 ingredients into medium bowl. Drizzle with olive oil. Sprinkle with next 3 ingredients. Toss until coated. Spread in single layer on greased baking sheet with sides. Bake for about 15 minutes until starting to brown.

Add tomatoes and garlic. Toss. Bake for another 5 minutes until tomatoes are hot and vegetables are tender-crisp. Add to quinoa. Toss.

Drizzle with remaining 3 ingredients. Toss until coated. Makes about 4 cups (1 L).

1/2 cup (125 mL): 161 Calories; 6.4 g Total Fat (4.1 g Mono, 1.0 g Poly, 0.8 g Sat); 0 mg Cholesterol; 23 g Carbohydrate; 2.4 g Fibre; 3.5 g Protein; 192 mg Sodium

CHOICES: 1 Grains & Starches; 1/2 Vegetables; 1 Fats

Spinach Feta Bulgur

Bulgur is livened up with spinach, feta, olives and a bright lemon finish. Fresh, flavourful and nutritious, too!

Canola oil	1 tsp.	5 mL
Chopped onion	1 cup	250 mL
Garlic cloves, minced, (or 1/2 tsp. 2 mL, powder)	2	2
Dried oregano	1/2 tsp.	2 mL
Pepper	1/4 tsp.	1 mL
Prepared vegetable broth	1 1/2 cups	375 mL
Bulgur	1/2 cup	125 mL
Fresh spinach leaves, lightly packed	4 cups	1 L
Crumbled light feta cheese	1/3 cup	75 mL
Sliced black olives	1/4 cup	60 mL
Grated lemon zest	1/2 tsp.	2 mL

Heat canola oil in large frying pan on medium. Add next 4 ingredients. Cook for about 5 minutes, stirring often, until onion is softened.

Add broth. Bring to a boil. Add bulgur. Stir. Boil gently, covered, for about 5 minutes, stirring occasionally, until bulgur is tender and broth is absorbed.

Add spinach. Heat and stir for about 2 minutes until wilted. Remove from heat.

Add remaining 3 ingredients. Stir. Makes about 3 cups (750 mL). Serves 4.

1 serving: 152 Calories; 4.7 g Total Fat (1.4 g Mono, 0.6 g Poly, 1.6 g Sat); 7 mg Cholesterol; 22 g Carbohydrate; 4 g Fibre; 8 g Protein; 524 mg Sodium

CHOICES: 1 Grains & Starches; 1/2 Meat & Alternatives

Rapid Ratatouille

Being in a hurry is no reason to settle for a second-rate side. This dish comes together quickly, and mixed vegetables have never tasted so good!

Chopped fresh basil	2 tbsp.	30 mL
(or 1 1/2 tsp., 7 mL, dried)		
Olive (or canola) oil	2 tbsp.	30 mL
Lemon juice	1 tbsp.	15 mL
Sweet chili sauce	1 tbsp.	15 mL
Garlic clove, minced	1	1
(or 1/4 tsp., 1 mL, powder)		
Salt	1/4 tsp.	1 mL
Pepper	1/4 tsp.	1 mL
Olive (or canola) oil	2 tsp.	10 mL
Sliced red pepper	2 cups	500 mL
Sliced Asian eggplant (with peel)	1 cup	250 mL
Sliced fresh white mushrooms	1 cup	250 mL
Sliced zucchini (with peel)	1 cup	250 mL

Combine first 7 ingredients in small bowl.

Heat wok or large frying pan on medium-high until very hot. Add second amount of olive oil. Add remaining 4 ingredients. Stir-fry for about 5 minutes until vegetables are tender-crisp. Add lemon juice mixture. Toss. Remove from heat. Let stand, covered, for 5 minutes to blend flavours. Makes about 4 cups (1 L). Serves 4.

1 serving: 130 Calories; 9.4 g Total Fat (6.7 g Mono, 1.0 g Poly, 1.3 g Sat); 0 mg Cholesterol; 12 g Carbohydrate; 4 g Fibre; 2 g Protein; 188 mg Sodium

CHOICES: 1 Vegetables; 1 Fats

Paré Pointer

A chicken lays an egg because if she dropped it, it would break.

Feta Ruby Chard

Introduce your family to this delicious and nutritious green with a simple sauté of chard, garlic and feta cheese.

Tub margarine	2 tsp.	10 mL
Sliced onion	1/2 cup	125 mL
Garlic clove, minced	1	1
(or 1/4 tsp., 1 mL, powder)		
Coarsely chopped ruby chard, lightly packed	9 cups	2.25 L
Prepared vegetable broth	2 tbsp.	30 mL
Crumbled feta cheese	1/4 cup	60 mL

Melt margarine in large saucepan on medium. Add onion and garlic. Cook, uncovered, for about 5 minutes, stirring often, until onion is softened and starting to brown.

Add chard and broth. Stir. Cook, covered, for about 4 minutes until chard starts to wilt. Stir. Cook for another 4 minutes until chard is wilted. Transfer to plate.

Sprinkle with cheese. Makes about 3 1/2 cups (875 mL). Serves 4.

1 serving: 66 Calories; 3.3 g Total Fat (0.9 g Mono, 0.8 g Poly, 1.1 g Sat); 4 mg Cholesterol; 7 g Carbohydrate; 2 g Fibre; 4 g Protein; 350 mg Sodium

CHOICES: 1 Vegetables

Pictured on front cover.

Creamy Polenta

This creamy polenta with hints of pepper and cheese is true comfort food. Try using it as a base for serving with stews or other saucy dishes.

Prepared vegetable broth	3 1/4 cups	800 mL
Yellow cornmeal	1 cup	250 mL
Grated Italian cheese blend	1/3 cup	75 mL
Coarsely ground pepper	1/2 tsp.	2 mL

(continued on next page)

138

Sides

Combine broth and cornmeal in 1.5 quart (1.5 L) casserole. Microwave, covered, on high (100%) for about 12 minutes, stirring every 3 minutes, until cornmeal is tender and broth is absorbed.

Add cheese and pepper. Stir. Makes about 4 cups (1 L). Serves 6.

1 serving: 123 Calories; 2.2 g Total Fat (0.1 g Mono, 0.2 g Poly, 1.1 g Sat); 4 mg Cholesterol; 21 g Carbohydrate; 2 g Fibre; 4 g Protein; 288 mg Sodium

CHOICES: 1 Grains & Starches

Edamame Succotash

Don't like lima beans? We've swapped them for a whole new legume in this familiar side. Edamame is high in protein and fibre and is a good source of vitamins and minerals. If you like, you could add a sprinkle of simulated bacon bits for a smoky flavour.

Canola oil	2 tsp.	10 mL
Chopped onion	1 cup	250 mL
Chopped red pepper	1/2 cup	125 mL
Garlic clove, minced	1	1
(or 1/4 tsp., 1 mL, powder)		
Can of diced tomatoes (with juice)	14 oz.	398 mL
Frozen kernel corn	1 1/2 cups	375 mL
Frozen shelled edamame (soybeans)	1 1/2 cups	375 mL
Prepared vegetable broth	1/4 cup	60 mL
Chili powder	2 tsp.	10 mL

Heat canola oil in large frying pan on medium. Add next 3 ingredients. Cook for about 5 minutes, stirring occasionally, until onion and red pepper start to soften.

Add remaining 5 ingredients. Bring to a boil. Reduce heat to medium-low. Cook, covered, for about 5 minutes, stirring occasionally, until edamame is tender-crisp. Makes about 4 cups (1 L). Serves 6.

1 serving: 119 Calories; 3.8 g Total Fat (0.9 g Mono, 0.6 g Poly, 0.3 g Sat); 0 mg Cholesterol; 17 g Carbohydrate; 3 g Fibre; 6 g Protein; 215 mg Sodium

CHOICES: 1/2 Grains & Starches; 1 Vegetables; 1/2 Meat & Alternatives

Ginger Biscuits
With Orange Cream

Finish a heavy meal with something sweet and light—delicate biscuits studded with crystallized ginger and served with a fresh orange-flavoured cream.

ORANGE CREAM

Can of mandarin orange segments, drained	10 oz.	285 g
Light sour cream	1/2 cup	125 mL
Frozen light whipped topping, thawed	1/2 cup	125 mL
Grated orange zest	1 tsp.	5 mL

GINGER BISCUITS

All-purpose flour	1 cup	250 mL
Whole-wheat flour	1/4 cup	60 mL
Granulated sugar	2 tbsp.	30 mL
Minced crystallized ginger	1 tsp.	5 mL
Baking powder	1/2 tsp.	2 mL
Baking soda	1/2 tsp.	2 mL
Ground ginger	1/2 tsp.	2 mL
Salt	1/4 tsp.	1 mL
Tub margarine	1/4 cup	60 mL
Large egg, fork-beaten	1	1
1% buttermilk	1/4 cup	60 mL

Orange Cream: Combine first 4 ingredients in small bowl. Chill for about 20 minutes. Makes about 2 cups (500 mL) cream.

Ginger Biscuits: Preheat oven to 425°F (220°C). Combine first 8 ingredients in medium bowl.

Cut in margarine until mixture resembles coarse crumbs.

Add egg and buttermilk. Stir until just moistened. Turn out onto lightly floured surface. Knead 4 or 5 times until dough just comes together. Roll out to 6 x 6 inch (15 x 15 cm) square. Transfer to greased baking sheet. Score 4 squares into dough, about 1/2 inch (12 mm) deep, using greased sharp knife. Cut each square into 2 triangles, for a total of 8 triangles. Bake for about 12 minutes until wooden pick inserted in centre comes out clean. Let stand on baking sheet for 5 minutes to cool. Makes 8 biscuits. Serve with Orange Cream.

(continued on next page)

*1 biscuit with 1/4 cup (60 mL) **Orange Cream:** 187 Calories; 8.2 g Total Fat (2.7 g Mono, 2.4 g Poly, 2.3 g Sat); 29 mg Cholesterol; 24 g Carbohydrate; 1 g Fibre; 4 g Protein; 272 mg Sodium*

CHOICES: 1 Grains & Starches; 1 1/2 Fats

Tropical Twist Iced Treat

What's the twist? This iced treat includes beans, which add protein and fibre, but the smooth, creamy texture will make you think you're eating soft-serve.

Canned navy beans, rinsed and drained	1 cup	250 mL
Orange juice	1/2 cup	125 mL
Package of fat-free instant white chocolate pudding powder (4-serving size)	1	1
Frozen mango pieces, chopped (do not thaw)	1 1/2 cups	375 mL
Frozen raspberries (do not thaw)	1 1/2 cups	375 mL

Process beans and orange juice in food processor, scraping down sides if necessary, until smooth.

Add pudding powder. Process until combined.

Add mango and raspberries. Process until smooth, scraping down sides if necessary. Serve immediately. Makes about 3 1/3 cups (825 mL). Serves 4.

*1 **serving:** 247 Calories; 0.9 g Total Fat (0.1 g Mono, 0.2 g Poly, 0.2 g Sat); 0 mg Cholesterol; 56 g Carbohydrate; 7 g Fibre; 6 g Protein; 444 mg Sodium*

CHOICES: 1/2 Grains & Starches; 1 Fruits; 1 1/2 Other Choices; 1/2 Meat & Alternatives

Chocolate Berry Parfaits

A light delight with layers of berries, chocolate pudding and creamy whipped topping.

Skim milk	2 cups	500 mL
Box of fat-free instant chocolate pudding powder (4-serving size)	1	1
Sliced fresh strawberries	1 cup	250 mL
Fresh blueberries	1 cup	250 mL
Frozen light whipped topping, thawed	1/4 cup	60 mL

Beat milk and pudding powder in small bowl for about 2 minutes until thickened. Chill for about 5 minutes until set.

Put strawberries into 4 tall glasses. Spoon half of pudding over strawberries. Scatter blueberries over pudding. Top with remaining pudding.

Spoon whipped topping over pudding. Makes 4 parfaits.

1 parfait: 193 Calories; 1.0 g Total Fat (0.1 g Mono, 0.1 g Poly, 0.7 g Sat); 2 mg Cholesterol; 43 g Carbohydrate; 2 g Fibre; 5 g Protein; 234 mg Sodium

CHOICES: 1/2 Fruits; 2 Other Choices; 1/2 Milk & Alternatives

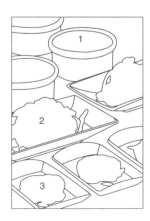

1. Berry Ricotta Custards, page 146
2. Triple-Chocolate Shortcakes, page 149
3. Crustless Cheesecake Bites, page 146

Props courtesy of: The Bay

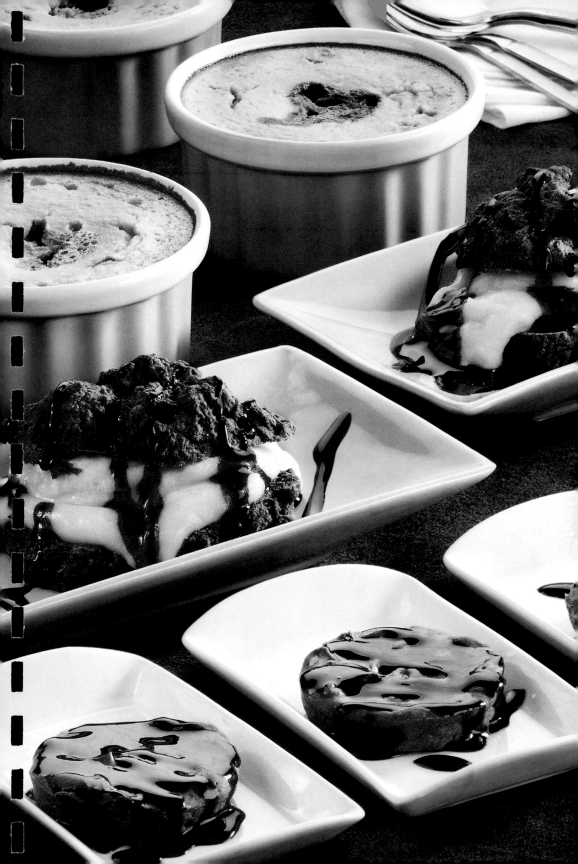

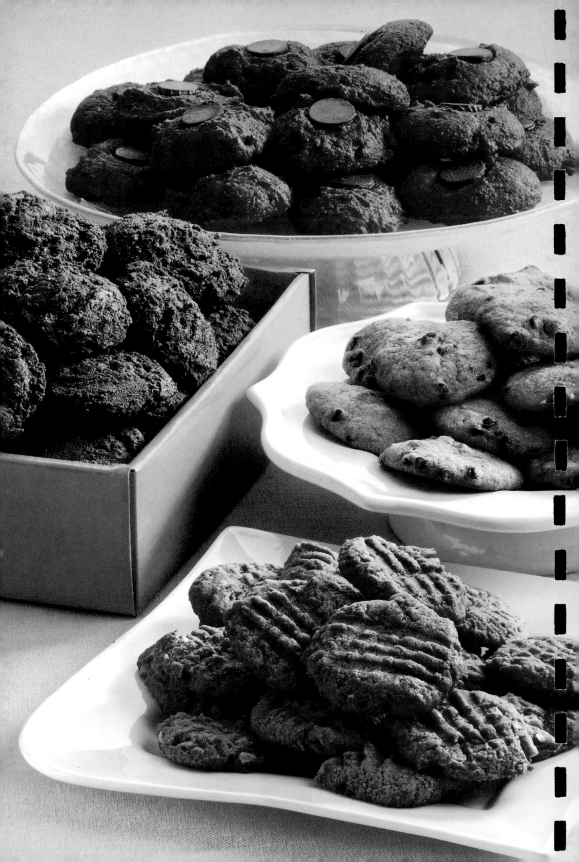

Grilled Peaches And Strawberries

Elegance can be this easy! The sweetness of grilled peaches and strawberries blend with the tanginess of honey and balsamic vinegar for the perfect combination.

Balsamic vinegar	1/4 cup	60 mL
Liquid honey	2 tbsp.	30 mL
Olive oil	2 tsp.	10 mL
Ground cinnamon	1/4 tsp.	1 mL
Ground ginger	1/2 tsp.	2 mL
Fresh peaches, halved and pitted	2	2
Large fresh strawberries	8	8

Preheat gas barbecue to medium-high. Whisk first 5 ingredients in large bowl.

Add peaches and strawberries. Toss until coated. Place peaches, cut-side down, on greased grill. Place strawberries on greased grill. Cook for about 6 minutes, turning once and brushing with vinegar mixture, until fruit is tender but firm. Transfer to 4 plates. Drizzle with remaining vinegar mixture. Serves 4.

1 serving: 97 Calories; 2.4 g Total Fat (1.7 g Mono, 0.3 g Poly, 0.3 g Sat); 0 mg Cholesterol; 19 g Carbohydrate; 2 g Fibre; 1 g Protein; 5 mg Sodium

CHOICES: 1/2 Fruits; 1/2 Other Choices; 1/2 Fats

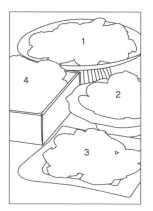

1. Pumpkin Power Puffs, page 51
2. Chocolate Chip Softies, page 47
3. Quick PB Cookies, page 59
4. Cocoa Coconut Macaroons, page 52

Desserts

Crustless Cheescake Bites

Craving cheesecake? These rich chocolate bites are loaded with cheesy goodness. This is one cheesecake you can indulge in, guilt-free!

95% fat-free cream cheese	8 oz.	250 g
Granulated sugar	1/3 cup	75 mL
All-purpose flour	2 tbsp.	30 mL
Cocoa powder, sifted if lumpy	1 tbsp.	15 mL
Large egg	1	1
Chocolate syrup	1/4 cup	60 mL

Preheat oven to 350°F (175°C). Beat first 4 ingredients in medium bowl until combined. Add egg. Beat until smooth. Divide into 12 greased muffin cups. Bake for about 12 minutes until set. Let stand in pan for 5 minutes. Carefully remove from pan and place on serving plate.

Drizzle with chocolate syrup. Makes 12 bites.

1 bite: 67 Calories; 0.7 g Total Fat (0.3 g Mono, 0.1 g Poly, 0.3 g Sat); 17 mg Cholesterol; 12 g Carbohydrate; trace Fibre; 4 g Protein; 112 mg Sodium

CHOICES: 1/2 Other Choices

Pictured on page 143.

Berry Ricotta Custards

Fresh berry flavour is complemented by light lemon in this comforting custard. Berry good!

Frozen mixed berries, thawed and drained	1 1/2 cups	375 mL
Large eggs	2	2
Light ricotta cheese	1 cup	250 mL
Granulated sugar	3 tbsp.	50 mL
Cornstarch	2 tbsp.	30 mL
Lemon juice	2 tsp.	10 mL
Grated lemon zest	1 tsp.	5 mL
Salt	1/8 tsp.	0.5 mL

(continued on next page)

Preheat oven to 400°F (205°C). Spoon berries into 4 greased 6 oz. (170 mL) ramekins.

Whisk remaining 7 ingredients in small bowl. Spoon over berries. Bake for about 20 minutes until knife inserted in centre of custard comes out clean. Makes 4 custards.

1 custard: 174 Calories; 5.0 g Total Fat (1.1 g Mono, 0.4 g Poly, 2.3 g Sat); 108 mg Cholesterol; 22 g Carbohydrate; 2 g Fibre; 8 g Protein; 159 mg Sodium

CHOICES: 1/2 Fruits; 1/2 Other Choices; 1 Meat & Alternatives

Pictured on page 143.

Blueberry Frozen Yogurt

Craving ice cream? This frosty frozen dessert combines the creaminess of pudding with the tanginess of yogurt and lemon—and it's virtually fat-free!

Box of fat-free instant vanilla pudding powder (4-serving size)	1	1
Non-fat plain yogurt	1 cup	250 mL
Frozen blueberries (do not thaw)	3 cups	750 mL
Lemon juice	1 tbsp.	15 mL

Process pudding powder and yogurt in food processor or blender for about 15 seconds, scraping down sides if necessary, until combined.

Add blueberries and lemon juice. Process, scraping down sides if necessary, until smooth. Spoon into 4 chilled dessert cups. Serve immediately. Makes about 2 1/2 cups (625 mL). Serves 4.

1 serving: 164 Calories; 0.8 g Total Fat (0 g Mono, 0 g Poly, trace Sat); 1 mg Cholesterol; 40 g Carbohydrate; 3 g Fibre; 3 g Protein; 172 mg Sodium

CHOICES: 1/2 Fruits; 1 1/2 Other Choices; 1/2 Milk & Alternatives

Strawberry Wafer Layers

Bring a little freshness to your dinner table with this layered dessert of sweet strawberry mousse and crisp cookie wafers.

WAFER COOKIES

Egg white (large), room temperature	1	1
Icing (confectioner's) sugar	1/4 cup	60 mL
All-purpose flour	2 1/2 tbsp.	37 mL
Tub margarine, melted	2 tbsp.	30 mL
Water	1 tsp.	5 mL
Vanilla extract	1/4 tsp.	1 mL

STRAWBERRY CREAM

Frozen fat-free whipped topping, thawed	1 1/2 cups	375 mL
Frozen sliced strawberries in light syrup, thawed (with syrup)	1/2 cup	125 mL
Frozen sliced strawberries in light syrup, thawed (with syrup)	1/2 cup	125 mL

Wafer Cookies: Preheat oven to 400°F (205°C). Whisk all 6 ingredients in small bowl until smooth. Spoon 8 portions of batter, using 2 tsp. (10 mL) for each, onto parchment paper-lined baking sheet. Spread to 3 inch (7.5 cm) circles. Bake for about 7 minutes until edges are browned and crisp. Transfer to wire rack to cool. Makes 8 cookies.

Strawberry Cream: Meanwhile, combine whipped topping and first amount of strawberries in small bowl. Makes about 2 cups (500 mL). Place 4 cookies on plates. Spoon half of strawberry mixture onto wafers. Repeat with remaining wafers and strawberry mixture.

Top with second amount of strawberries. Serves 4.

1 serving: 179 Calories; 5.8 g Total Fat (2.4 g Mono, 2.3 g Poly, 0.8 g Sat); 0 mg Cholesterol; 29 g Carbohydrate; trace Fibre; 2 g Protein; 106 mg Sodium

CHOICES: 1/2 Fruits; 1/2 Other Choices; 1 Fats

Pictured on page 108.

Triple-Chocolate Shortcakes

Three times the chocolate! Light-flavoured chocolate biscuits are filled with white chocolate pudding and topped with a dark chocolate drizzle.

All-purpose flour	1 1/4 cups	300 mL
Brown sugar, packed	3 tbsp.	50 mL
Cocoa powder, sifted if lumpy	2 tbsp.	30 mL
Baking powder	1 tsp.	5 mL
Baking soda	1/4 tsp.	1 mL
Salt	1/8 tsp.	0.5 mL
Tub margarine	2 tbsp.	30 mL
1% buttermilk	1/2 cup	125 mL
Vanilla extract	1 tsp.	5 mL
Box of fat-free instant white chocolate pudding powder (4-serving size)	1	1
Skim milk	2 cups	500 mL
Chocolate syrup	2 tbsp.	30 mL

Preheat oven to 450°F (230°C). Combine first 6 ingredients in large bowl. Cut in margarine until mixture resembles coarse crumbs.

Add buttermilk and vanilla. Stir until just moistened. Drop 6 portions of batter, using 3 tbsp. (50 mL) for each, about 2 inches (5 cm) apart onto greased baking sheet. Bake for about 10 minutes until wooden pick inserted in centre of biscuit comes out clean. Transfer to wire rack to cool slightly.

Meanwhile, beat pudding powder and milk in small bowl for about 2 minutes until thickened. Chill for about 5 minutes until set. Cut biscuits in half horizontally. Transfer to plates. Spoon about 1/4 cup (60 mL) pudding onto each biscuit bottom. Set biscuit tops over pudding. Spoon 1 tbsp. (15 mL) pudding over top of each.

Drizzle with chocolate syrup. Makes 6 shortcakes.

1 shortcake: 275 Calories; 4.4 g Total Fat (1.7 g Mono, 1.5 g Poly, 0.9 g Sat); 3 mg Cholesterol; 53 g Carbohydrate; 1 g Fibre; 7 g Protein; 381 mg Sodium

CHOICES: 1 Grains & Starches; 2 Other Choices; 1/2 Milk & Alternatives; 1 Fats

Pictured on page 143.

Measurement Tables

Throughout this book measurements are given in Conventional and Metric measure. To compensate for differences between the two measurements due to rounding, a full metric measure is not always used. The cup used is the standard 8 fluid ounce. Temperature is given in degrees Fahrenheit and Celsius. Baking pan measurements are in inches and centimetres as well as quarts and litres. An exact metric conversion is given below as well as the working equivalent (Metric Standard Measure).

Spoons

Conventional Measure	Metric Exact Conversion Millilitre (mL)	Metric Standard Measure Millilitre (mL)
1/8 teaspoon (tsp.)	0.6 mL	0.5 mL
1/4 teaspoon (tsp.)	1.2 mL	1 mL
1/2 teaspoon (tsp.)	2.4 mL	2 mL
1 teaspoon (tsp.)	4.7 mL	5 mL
2 teaspoons (tsp.)	9.4 mL	10 mL
1 tablespoon (tbsp.)	14.2 mL	15 mL

Cups

Conventional Measure	Metric Exact Conversion Millilitre (mL)	Metric Standard Measure Millilitre (mL)
1/4 cup (4 tbsp.)	56.8 mL	60 mL
1/3 cup (5 1/3 tbsp.)	75.6 mL	75 mL
1/2 cup (8 tbsp.)	113.7 mL	125 mL
2/3 cup (10 2/3 tbsp.)	151.2 mL	150 mL
3/4 cup (12 tbsp.)	170.5 mL	175 mL
1 cup (16 tbsp.)	227.3 mL	250 mL
4 1/2 cups	1022.9 mL	1000 mL (1 L)

Oven Temperatures

Fahrenheit (°F)	Celsius (°C)
175°	80°
200°	95°
225°	110°
250°	120°
275°	140°
300°	150°
325°	160°
350°	175°
375°	190°
400°	205°
425°	220°
450°	230°
475°	240°
500°	260°

Dry Measurements

Conventional Measure Ounces (oz.)	Metric Exact Conversion Grams (g)	Metric Standard Measure Grams (g)
1 oz.	28.3 g	28 g
2 oz.	56.7 g	57 g
3 oz.	85.0 g	85 g
4 oz.	113.4 g	125 g
5 oz.	141.7 g	140 g
6 oz.	170.1 g	170 g
7 oz.	198.4 g	200 g
8 oz.	226.8 g	250 g
16 oz.	453.6 g	500 g
32 oz.	907.2 g	1000 g (1 kg)

Pans

Conventional Inches	Metric Centimetres
8x8 inch	20x20 cm
9x9 inch	22x22 cm
9x13 inch	22x33 cm
10x15 inch	25x38 cm
11x17 inch	28x43 cm
8x2 inch round	20x5 cm
9x2 inch round	22x5 cm
10x4 1/2 inch tube	25x11 cm
8x4x3 inch loaf	20x10x7.5 cm
9x5x3 inch loaf	22x12.5x7.5 cm

Casseroles

CANADA & BRITAIN Standard Size Casserole	Exact Metric Measure	UNITED STATES Standard Size Casserole	Exact Metric Measure
1 qt. (5 cups)	1.13 L	1 qt. (4 cups)	900 mL
1 1/2 qts. (7 1/2 cups)	1.69 L	1 1/2 qts. (6 cups)	1.35 L
2 qts. (10 cups)	2.25 L	2 qts. (8 cups)	1.8 L
2 1/2 qts. (12 1/2 cups)	2.81 L	2 1/2 qts. (10 cups)	2.25 L
3 qts. (15 cups)	3.38 L	3 qts. (12 cups)	2.7 L
4 qts. (20 cups)	4.5 L	4 qts. (16 cups)	3.6 L
5 qts. (25 cups)	5.63 L	5 qts. (20 cups)	4.5 L

Recipe Index

151

152

153

154

155

156

Company's Coming cookbooks are available at retail locations throughout Canada!

EXCLUSIVE mail order offer on next page

Buy any 2 cookbooks—choose a 3rd FREE of equal or lesser value than the lowest price paid.

Original Series $15.99

CODE		CODE		CODE	
SQ	150 Delicious Squares	CCLFC	Low-Fat Cooking	GBR	Ground Beef Recipes
CA	Casseroles	SCH	Stews, Chilies & Chowders	FRIR	4-Ingredient Recipes
MU	Muffins & More	FD	Fondues	KHC	Kids' Healthy Cooking
SA	Salads	CCBE	The Beef Book	MM	Mostly Muffins
AP	Appetizers	RC	The Rookie Cook	SP	Soups
CO	Cookies	RHR	Rush-Hour Recipes	SU	Simple Suppers
PA	Pasta	SW	Sweet Cravings	CCDC	Diabetic Cooking
BA	Barbecues	YRG	Year-Round Grilling	CHN	Chicken Now
PR	Preserves	GG	Garden Greens	KDS	Kids Do Snacks
CH	Chicken, Etc.	CHC	Chinese Cooking	TMRC	30-Minute Rookie Cook
CT	Cooking For Two	BEV	The Beverage Book	LFE	Low-Fat Express
SC	Slow Cooker Recipes	SCD	Slow Cooker Dinners	SI	Choosing Sides
SF	Stir-Fry	WM	30-Minute Weekday Meals	PAS	Perfect Pasta And Sauces
MAM	Make-Ahead Meals	SDL	School Days Lunches	TMDC	30-Minute Diabetic Cooking
PB	The Potato Book	PD	Potluck Dishes		**NEW** Oct. 15/08

Cookbook Author Biography

CODE	$15.99
JP	Jean Paré: An Appetite for Life

Most Loved Recipe Collection

CODE	$23.99
MLBQ	Most Loved Barbecuing

CODE	$24.99
MLSD	Most Loved Salads & Dressings
MLCA	Most Loved Casseroles
MLSF	Most Loved Stir-Fries
MLHF	Most Loved Holiday Favourites
MLSC	Most Loved Slow Cooker Creations
MLDE	Most Loved Summertime Desserts **NEW** April 1/08

3-in-1 Cookbook Collection

CODE	$29.99
MME	Meals Made Easy **NEW** June 1/08

2-in-1 Cookbook Collection

CODE	$24.99
HECH	Healthy Choices

Lifestyle Series

CODE	$19.99
DDI	Diabetic Dinners
HH	Healthy in a Hurry
WGR	Whole Grain Recipes

Special Occasion Series

CODE	$24.99
CGFK	Christmas Gifts from the Kitchen
TR	Timeless Recipes for All Occasions
CCT	Company's Coming–Tonight! **NEW** Oct. 1/08

CODE	$27.99
CCEL	Christmas Celebrations

CODE	$29.99
CATH	Cooking At Home

Practical Gourmet – NEW!

CODE	$29.99
SPFS	Small Plates for Sharing **NEW** Sept. 1/08

157

Order **ONLINE** for fast delivery!

Log onto **www.companyscoming.com**, browse through our library of cookbooks, gift sets and newest releases and place your order using our fast and secure online order form.

TITLE	CODE	QUANTITY	PRICE	TOTAL
			$	$

DON'T FORGET to indicate your FREE BOOK(S). (see exclusive mail order offer above) PLEASE PRINT

TOTAL BOOKS (including FREE)

TOTAL BOOKS PURCHASED

	INTERNATIONAL via Air Mail	USA	Canada
Shipping & Handling First Book (per destination)	$32.98 (one book)	$9.98 (one book)	$5.98 (one book)
Additional Books (include FREE books)	$ ($7.99 each)	$ ($1.99 each)	$ ($1.99 each)
Sub-Total	$	$	$
Canadian residents add GST/HST			$
TOTAL AMOUNT ENCLOSED	$	$	$

Terms

- All orders must be prepaid. Sorry, no CODs.
- Canadian orders are processed in Canadian funds. US International orders. are processed in US Funds.
- Prices are subject to change without prior notice.
- Canadian residents must pay GST/HST (no provincial tax required).
- No tax is required for orders outside Canada.
- Satisfaction is guaranteed or return within 30 days for a full refund.
- Make cheque or money order payable to: **Company's Coming Publishing Limited** 2311-96 Street, Edmonton, Alberta Canada T6N 1G3.
- Orders are shipped surface mail. For courier rates, visit our website: **www.companyscoming.com** or contact us: **Tel: 780-450-6223 Fax: 780-450-1857.**

Gift Giving

- Let us help you with your gift giving!
- We will send cookbooks directly to the recipients of your choice if you give us their names and addresses.
- Please specify the titles you wish to send to each person.
- If you would like to include a personal note or card, we will be pleased to enclose it with your gift order.
- Company's Coming Cookbooks make excellent gifts: birthdays, bridal showers, Mother's Day, Father's Day, graduation or any occasion ...collect them all!

□ MasterCard □ VISA Expiry ___ / ___ MO/YR

Credit Card # _____

Name of cardholder _____

Cardholder signature _____

Shipping Address Send the cookbooks listed above to:

□ **Please check if this is a Gift Order**

Name: _____

Street: _____

City: _____ Prov./State: _____

Postal Code/Zip: _____ Country: _____

Tel: (___) _____

E-mail address: _____

Your privacy is important to us. We will not share your e-mail address or personal information with any outside party.

□ **YES! Please add me to your News Bite e-mail newsletter.**

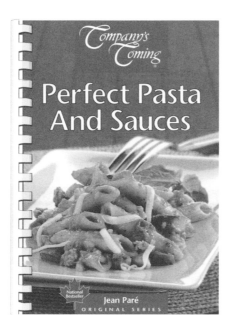

Perfect Pasta And Sauces

Jean Paré
ORIGINAL SERIES

Whether you're starting from scratch or with a box of pasta, these all-new recipes have the pasta lover in mind—and with a separate sauce section, the pastabilities are endless!

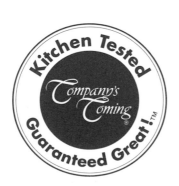

Kitchen Tested
Company's Coming
Guaranteed Great!™

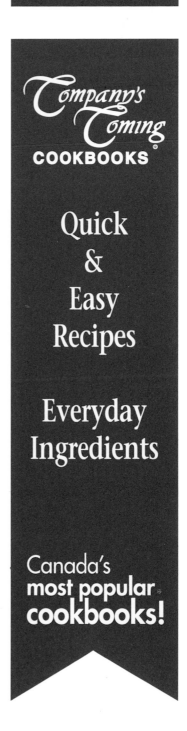

Cookmark

Company's Coming
COOKBOOKS®

Quick & Easy Recipes

Everyday Ingredients

Canada's **most popular** cookbooks!